hair savers
for women

OTHER BOOKS BY THE AUTHOR

Natural Weight Loss Miracles
21 Days to Better Fitness
Kava: The Ultimate Guide to Nature's Anti-Stress Herb
The Cellulite Breakthrough

OTHER BOOKS COAUTHORED BY THE AUTHOR

Lean Bodies
Lean Bodies Total Fitness
30 Days to Swimsuit Lean
High Performance Nutrition
Power Eating
Shape Training
High Performance Bodybuilding
50 Workout Secrets
BUILT! The New Bodybuilding for Everyone

hair savers
for women

A COMPLETE
GUIDE TO
PREVENTING
AND TREATING
HAIR LOSS

MAGGIE GREENWOOD-ROBINSON, Ph.D.

THREE RIVERS PRESS
NEW YORK

The suggestions for usage of prescription medicines, nonprescription products, hair-care products, surgical and nonsurgical procedures, nutritional and herbal supplements, and other hair-loss treatments are not intended to replace medical advice or treatment by your physician. All questions and concerns regarding your hair loss and other medical conditions should be directed toward your physician or dermatologist.

Long-term use of nutritional supplements is not recommended unless it is done under the guidance and supervision of a physician. Please consult your physician prior to supplementing with herbs and other supplements or using nonprescription hair care products.

All attempts have been made to include the most recent and factual research and medical reports about hair-loss treatments. However, there is no guarantee that future studies will not change the recommendations and information presented here.

The mention of specific products or brands in this book does not constitute an endorsement by either the author or the publisher.

Published by Three Rivers Press, New York, New York.
Member of the Crown Publishing Group.

Random House, Inc. New York, Toronto, London, Sydney, Auckland
www.randomhouse.com

THREE RIVERS PRESS is a registered trademark and the Three Rivers Press colophon is a trademark of Random House, Inc.

Printed in the United States of America

Design by Maggie Hinders

Library of Congress Cataloging-in-Publication Data

Greenwood-Robinson, Maggie.
    Hair savers for women : a complete guide to preventing and
treating hair loss / by Maggie Greenwood-Robinson.
        p.   cm.
    Includes bibliographical references (p.).
    1. Baldness.   2. Women—Health and hygiene.   I. Title.
    RL155.G74   2000
    616.5'46—dc21   99-39185
                                                        CIP

ISBN 0-609-80445-6

To my husband Jeff, with love.

Contents

Acknowledgments

I gratefully thank the following people for their work and contributions to this book: Madeleine Morel, 2M Communications, Ltd.; Sarah Silbert, PJ Dempsey and Elizabeth Bird, The Crown Publishing Group; Wilma Bergfeld, M.D., F.A.C.P., head of Dermatology, Clinical Research and Dermatopathology at the Cleveland Clinic; Jean-Claude Bystryn, M.D., Professor of Dermatology, New York University School of Medicine; Dr. Emily A. Kane, N.D., L.Ac., Doctor of Naturopathic Medicine; and Philip Kingsley, Consultant Trichologist, Philip Kingsley Trichological Centre.

Introduction

U NLIKE OSTEOPOROSIS, PMS, menopause, or other female disorders, women's hair loss is rarely talked about. Yet more than 20 million women in the United States suffer from a heredity type of baldness, and millions more are losing their hair as a result of medical and psychological causes.

Despite the prevalence of the problem, women have very little information on how to prevent, treat, and reverse baldness, most likely because hair loss has long been considered a male problem.

If you are suffering from hair loss, you have no doubt felt the frustration of not knowing what to do—a frustration compounded by the psychological impact of losing your hair. But no longer can the problem be ignored, or talked about in hushed tones. Women's hair loss must be addressed in a solution-oriented fashion so that the millions who suffer from it can gain sorely needed hope.

Thus, in *Hair Savers*, I have attempted to bring you the very latest solutions and advances in treating hair loss, from conventional medicine to natural remedies, and introduce you to a whole new world of safe, clinically proven baldness remedies. Also featured in *Hair Savers* are recommendations from leading authorities, including medical doctors, on how to treat your hair loss.

Some of treatments covered in *Hair Savers* fall into the category of alternative medicine. They may appear interesting but seem unusual. Yet they may be worth a try, particularly those backed by scientific research. Medical science is slowly learning that the most effective treatments are those that combine conventional medicine with alternative medicine.

Much of the information in this book is cutting edge, thanks to an ever-expanding base of research on treating hair loss. Armed with this knowledge, you'll be empowered to make informed choices about which course of treatment to pursue—and in so doing, save your hair and "get growing" again.

PART I

All About Hair and Hair Loss

ONE

Hair Today, Gone Tomorrow

THE SHOCK sets in when you find your shower drain clogged with hair . . . or your pillow covered with scads of loose hairs.

Could it be that you're losing your hair? It's hard to believe—that only happens to men, or does it? Although hair loss is not generally associated with women, it's a significant, serious, and widespread female health problem—one that causes embarrassment, frustration, depression, anxiety, poor self-esteem, even marriage problems. It can make you feel older and more self-conscious, too, plus you tend to worry excessively about how to conceal your hair loss.

What's more, hair loss in women is a "closet problem." No one likes to talk about it, and until only recently, there was very little information available on how to treat it.

Let's face it: Hair loss is traumatic. Bald is definitely not beautiful for women!

If your once-thick hair is falling out in clumps, or if you've got bald patches peeking out from your scalp, you're not alone. More than 20 million women in the United States alone—40 percent of them under age forty—are suffering from hair loss.

If your hair has started to thin out, take heart. You can do something about it. There are more options available than ever before to prevent and treat hair loss. A vast number of prescription medications have been scientifically shown to slow down, even reverse, hair loss. Newer, over-the-counter potions offer hope, too, when before there was none. What's more, huge advances have been made in surgical procedures, such as hair transplantation and scalp reduction, to help restore your hair to its former crowning glory. This is an exciting time in the treatment of hair loss!

Educate Yourself About Hair Loss

If you're suffering from hair loss, one of the most important moves you can make now is to investigate your condition. It's vital that you understand as much as you can about all the possible treatments available—and take responsibility for your own care. That way, you can be proactive in seeking solutions and participating in the management of your treatment. Reading this book is a good first step, especially since it's the first comprehensive look at hair loss in women—and how to treat it.

Choose Your Dermatologist Wisely

It is vital to seek a qualified dermatologist to treat your condition. A dermatologist is a physician who specializes in the treatment of skin diseases, including hair loss and baldness. Find one who understands the problem of hair in women, is sympathetic, and will support your desire to try various treatments. Talking to other women, contacting your local medical society, investigating a dermatologist's credentials, and interviewing the physician personally will help you decide whether to enlist that particular doctor's services.

As you search for a dermatologist, look for one who:
- Has special expertise in treating hair loss in women.
- Is board-certified in dermatology. Board certification indicates that a physician is exceptionally qualified in his or her field of medicine.

- Is genuinely interested in your symptoms and case.
- Is open to pursuing alternative medical options.

You may also want to consider a female physician. Often, but not always, women doctors offer emotional support more freely than male doctors do. Plus, you may feel more comfortable talking about your hair loss with another woman.

Unfortunately though, if you are enrolled in a health maintenance organization (HMO), you may not have the freedom of choice in selecting a dermatologist. If that's the case, you must tactfully motivate your HMO dermatologist to work with you to treat your condition.

If your hair loss does not respond to medication, you may want to consider undergoing the procedure known as a hair transplant. If so, you will have to consult a good hair transplantation surgeon. Guidelines for selecting a qualified surgeon are found on pages 200–201.

Hair Loss and Alternative Medicine

More than ever, people are turning to alternative medicine for disease prevention and treatment. A study recently published in the *Journal of the American Medical Association* reported that four out of every ten Americans used alternative therapies in 1997. And, according to another recent survey, approximately 60 percent of households view alternative medicine as complementary to conventional medicine.

Alternative medicine includes such therapies as acupuncture, chiropractic care, nutrition, herbalism, yoga, massage, hypnotherapy, and relaxation techniques. Increasingly, alternative medicine is being used as supportive treatment for certain kinds of hair loss. Nondrug products, nutrition, supplements, herbs, and natural hair care products are among the alternative medicine options discussed in this book.

If you're using or considering alternative medicine, discuss your decision with your physician. Tell him or her what you're using, why you're using it, and how it's working. That way, your alternative care can be coordinated with the conventional care you are receiving from your physician.

Many women are afraid to discuss alternative medicine with their physicians for fear they'll brush off or pooh-pooh the decision. But this isn't always the case. More physicians today are open to alternative therapies—and are employing them in their own practices. They realize that the benefits of alternative medicine are too overwhelming to ignore. In fact, the National Institutes of Health (NIH) has already funded more than seventy studies on various types of alternative medicine. And nearly half the medical schools in the United States are offering courses on alternative medicine. More good news: Many health care plans now cover alternative treatments.

If your doctor is opposed to your use of alternative remedies, find out why. It could be that the treatment is medically unsafe and harmful to your health, based on your medical history. Some herbs, for example, interact dangerously with prescription medication, or can aggravate existing health problems.

In some cases, doctors are simply uninformed about certain alternative therapies. One reason is that they don't have time to sift through all the data. Providing medical research you've uncovered on your own may help educate your doctor.

Suppose your doctor isn't open to alternative care, can't give a specific reason for his or her opposition, or seems to put down your decision. What next?

Consider finding another health care provider—someone who can incorporate the best of conventional medicine with the best of alternative care to give you the greatest overall chance for reversing your hair loss.

TWO

The Thick
and Thin of Hair

H AIR. We comb it, color it, curl it, twist it, tie it, or braid it. We may spend hours at a hair salon, or in front of a mirror trying to get it to look just right. When it does, we feel terrific. When it doesn't, we're down and distraught. Sometimes, a "bad hair day" can feel like the end of the world.

According to a recent survey, conducted by the cosmetic company Helene Curtis, 83 percent of the women polled said their hair strongly influences how they feel about themselves.

Hair has enormous power over our psyche—power we give it. This is because hair is an adornment, one of the main ways we make ourselves look pretty. Hair enhances beauty, and can let us make statements about our individuality.

Practically though, the real job of hair is to protect the body—against heat loss to keep us warm and against the potentially harmful rays of the sun. Were it not for hair, we might become deathly ill. Certain proteins in the brain are quite vulnerable to the sun's rays. Unless the scalp is shielded by hair, sun exposure can harm the brain and lead to sunstroke. Thus, hair performs some very useful functions. It's truly an amazing yet complex part of the human body.

The Anatomy of Hair

Trips to the hair salon every six weeks or so are visible proof that your hair grows rather steadily—something we take for granted. But if you zoomed down to the microscopic level of your scalp, you'd be amazed at how complex the process really is.

Hair emerges from the *follicle*, a hollow, sacklike pocket just below the surface of the scalp. In the womb, hair follicles appear when a developing fetus is nine weeks old.

On average, there are about 100,000 follicles on your scalp. The exact number and distribution is determined by your genes. The more follicles you have, and the more tightly packed they are, the denser your hair will be. Each individual follicle exerts control over the hair growing out of it.

Hair is made from a tough but elastic protein known as *keratin*, the same substance found in your fingernails and toenails. Keratin is produced by cells known as *keratinocytes* and forms nearly 97 percent of the hair shaft. The remaining 3 percent of your hair is moisture.

Remarkably, hair and its follicles are among the few parts of your body that repeatedly die and regenerate throughout your life span. In some ways, hair growth resembles tumor growth. That's why cancer specialists are studying the cellular controls of the hair follicle to see if it will give up some of its secrets—secrets that might help find a cure for cancer.

At the base of the follicle is the part of hair called the *root*. The root balloons into a soft bulblike structure called the *dermal papilla*, a group of specialized cells that orchestrate hair growth. If the dermal papilla is large, with lots of cells, the hair emerging from that follicle will be very thick.

Enveloping the dermal papilla is a region of cells known as the *matrix*. Hair is produced from the rapidly dividing cells of the matrix.

Tiny blood vessels at the base of the follicle feed it with nutrients to support hair growth. Healthy hair growth requires a constant supply of vitamins, minerals, and amino acids (protein

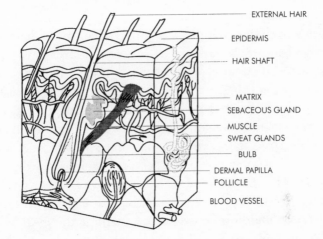

EXTERNAL HAIR
EPIDERMIS
HAIR SHAFT
MATRIX
SEBACEOUS GLAND
MUSCLE
SWEAT GLANDS
BULB
DERMAL PAPILLA
FOLLICLE
BLOOD VESSEL

Figure 2-1 Anatomy of Hair

particles) so that the follicle can manufacture new hair. Also at the base of the follicle are sensitive nerve endings called *dendrites* that reach into the follicles, which is why plucking out your hair often causes pain.

Near the follicles are tiny *sebaceous glands* that keep your hair lubricated and shiny. Connected to the follicles by short ducts, these glands manufacture a yellowish, oily secretion called *sebum* that can absorb and lock in large amounts of moisture. Sebum is a mixture of fats, cholesterol, proteins, and salts. When sebum is in short supply, your scalp turns dry and scaly, and your hair may break or split. Too much sebum, however, has been associated with hair loss.

There are also muscles called *erector pili* attached to each hair follicle. These muscles contract when you're cold or afraid. It is this same contraction that makes an animal's hair go vertical in response to fright, or causes goose bumps on human skin.

Interestingly, hair first moves downward into the follicle as it begins to grow, but after a few days, it is pushed back up. By the time hair becomes visible above the skin, it is actually nonliving tissue, composed of dead keratin cells. These dead protein cells are woven together like a tiny rope to form the hair strand. Each strand has three layers. The outermost layer is the *cuticle*, constructed of tightly packed, overlapping cells that resemble the scales on a fish. The cuticle protects your hair against water loss but can be easily damaged by heat, sun, chemicals, or overtreatment (such as blow-drying, perming, or bleaching). Forming the bulk of the hair strand is the *cortex*, which gives your hair its strength. Hair is as strong as a piece of wire and will rip apart only after it has been stretched by as much as 70 percent. The cortex also determines whether your hair is straight or curly.

The innermost center of the strand is the *medulla*. Its duty is not well understood, although its ability to reflect light gives your hair its sheen and variations in color tone.

Cells called *melanocytes* located near the base of the follicle make the pigment that determines hair color. Two kinds of pigment produce hair color. *Eumelanin* gives hair a brown to black color, and *pheomelanin* is responsible for blond and red shades. Varying concentrations of these pigments influence how light or dark your hair is. To provide color, melanocytes enter the hair fiber just as it is being developed during cell division. When melanocytes stop making pigment, your hair turns gray. Gray hair tends to run in families, but it is also related to aging and sometimes to stress.

There are ethnic differences in hair, too. Generally, Asians have the thickest and coarsest hair, compared to other ethnic groups, with more follicles on their scalps. In addition, Asian hair is always straight and very dark. African Americans have hair that is dark, curly, and coarse. Among Caucasians, you find the widest variability in hair density, thickness, and color.

Human Hair

There are three types of human hair. *Lanugo* is the fine, soft, colorless hair that covers an unborn baby and is shed at about the eighth month of fetal development. *Vellus* (from the Latin word for "fleece") is the soft, fluffy postnatal hair that remains on the entire body, except for the palms of the hands, soles of the feet, and other normally hairless portions. As a baby grows, vellus hair gradually turns into *terminal hair*, the coarser, pigmented hair that appears on the scalp, face, armpits, and pubic areas. Also called *nonvellus hair*, terminal hair on the scalp grows in a clockwise whorl pattern from the top of the head. The hair around your face grows in an angled direction away from your forehead and temples.

The hair follicle can switch from producing vellus hair to terminal hair and back again. You experience this during puberty when the hair follicles around your genitals and armpits convert from making vellus hair to making terminal hair. Likewise, the follicles can switch from producing terminal hair to making vellus hair—a reversal that occurs in certain types of hair loss.

No new hair follicles are formed after birth. So what you're born with, you have for life. From those follicles grow roughly 5 million hairs, covering your entire body. Under normal conditions, about 100,000 of them are found on your scalp. However, natural blonds have more hair (140,000) than brunettes (105,000) or redheads (90,000). (See Table 2-1 on page 12 for other fascinating facts about hair.)

Phases of Growth

You may think your hair grows every day, but it doesn't. Hair goes through phases of growth and rest.

The active growth phase is technically known as *anagen*. During this phase, cells in the dermal papilla enlarge, and the cells in the matrix undergo rapid division, ultimately sprouting new hair and allowing your hair to grow in length. On average, hair grows about six inches a year, and if left uncut, can reach a maximum of two and a half feet in length, depending on your hair's individual, genetically programmed growing cycle. The anagen phase lasts about three years, although this varies from person to person. A woman's scalp hair grows faster than a man's does.

Table 2-1. Fascinating Facts About Hair

- Hair protects your body from heat, cold, and the rays of the sun.
- The adult human scalp averages about 100,000 hairs.
- About 50 to 150 hairs are normally shed every day, or more than 4 million by age sixty.
- Hair on your scalp grows for two to five years, then rests for about three months.
- At any given time, about 10 percent of the hair on your head is in its resting phase.
- Hair grows about half an inch a month, or about six inches a year.
- If left uncut, hair can grow to a maximum of two and a half feet in length.
- If you never cut your hair, it would stop growing after about three years.
- Hair grows fastest in the summer and slowest in the winter.
- Female scalp hair grows faster than male scalp hair.
- The shape of hair follicles determines the type of hair. Straight hair comes from round follicles; wavy hair from oval follicles; and curly hair from flat follicles.
- Your hair is thickest at about the age of twenty. Hair thickness continues to shrink after that and becomes as fine as baby hair by age seventy.
- Hair thinning starts becoming noticeable only after about 40 percent of your hair has been lost.

The energy to drive the cell division that takes place during anagen comes from fat and glycogen, which is essentially a type of carbohydrate stored by the body for fuel. Follicles are also rich in DNA and RNA, nucleic acids that carry genetic information.

Following the anagen phase, the follicle enters *catagen*, a short transitional period lasting just a few days to as long as three weeks. During catagen, cell division grinds to a halt and finally stops altogether.

The follicle then enters *telogen*, the name given to the resting phase of the growth cycle. Basically, the hair stops growing but remains anchored in the follicle until it is shed or plucked. Hair that sits in the resting follicle is called a *club hair*.

You naturally shed 50 to 150 hairs daily, or more than 4 million by the time you reach age sixty. Telogen usually lasts about three months and can be compared to the molting you see in your dog or cat. At any given time, about 10 percent of the hair on your head is in the telogen phase. It is believed that telogen is partly under hormonal control.

After telogen, hair is pushed out of the way, or shed, to make room for a new hair, which then grows from the same follicle. Typically, this hair is a clone of the previous one. But the older you get, the less of a clone it is. With age, each new strand of hair becomes finer.

Hair growth is also affected by the season of the year. In the summer and spring, for example, hair grows very rapidly. You start shedding the most hair in the fall, peaking in November, and further fallout occurs in the spring.

Under normal circumstances, hair growth follows this distinct pattern of rest and activity. But sometimes its life cycle becomes disrupted, and you begin losing hair with alarming frequency—and in abnormal clumps. There are many reasons why women in all stages of life begin to lose their hair. Learning all you can about the cause of your hair loss is the first step toward treating it, and reversing its course.

THREE

Unlocking the Mystery of Hair Loss

Y OUR HAIR is falling out and you don't know why. The reason could be as simple as an iron deficiency or as complex as a hormonal problem. Understanding the possible causes, and identifying them early, can help you seek the right treatment—treatment that can potentially alter the course of your hair loss and save your hair from further shedding.

Alopecia

Medically, hair loss, or balding, is called "alopecia," which means "fox" in Greek. The Greek philosopher Aristotle noticed that foxes developed bare patches from mange, and so he described baldness as alopecia.

The various types of alopecia are discussed below and listed in order of the most common to the least common. Following each discussion is a list of symptoms, treatments, alternative therapies, and surgical and nonsurgical hair restoration options—all described in detail elsewhere in this book.

ANDROGENETIC ALOPECIA (HEREDITARY HAIR LOSS)

The most common cause of hair loss is rooted in your genes. Known technically as *androgenetic alopecia*, hereditary hair loss can begin any time after puberty, but usually sets in before the age of forty and may accelerate around the time you reach menopause.

Androgenetic alopecia affects both men and women. Balding men typically get receding hair lines and large patches of hair loss fringed by a horseshoe-shaped ruffle of hair, whereas women generally have diffuse hair thinning all over the scalp, most noticeably over the top of the scalp, just behind the bangs. About 50 percent of all women who experience hair loss have androgenetic alopecia, also termed *female-pattern baldness*.

If your hair is vanishing, you may have inherited the gene for hair loss, but not necessarily from your mom. This gene can come from either parent.

As a result of genetics, cells in hair follicles become abnormally sensitive to certain hormones. Like a telephone line, these hormones transmit messages that tell the follicle to produce less hair. In response, those follicles express their genetic fate by shortening their growing cycles and making thinner and finer hair. Some follicles go on permanent strike, stopping production altogether. Thus, androgenetic alopecia involves both genetic and hormonal factors.

The hormones that affect hair loss are known collectively as *androgens*. In women, androgens are produced by the ovaries and adrenal glands.

Two common androgens are testosterone, found in higher concentrations in men than in women, and DHEA (dehydroepi-androterone). These androgens constantly bathe the hair follicles.

Cells in the follicles contain enzymes known as *5 alpha-reductase*, of which there are two types, *5 alpha-reductase type 1* and *5 alpha-reductase type 2*. Type 1 is located mainly in the sebaceous glands, dermal papilla cells, and sweat glands. Type 2 is found primarily in the root of the hair follicle. Women with androgenetic alopecia have higher levels of 5 alpha-reductase enzymes, especially in the hair follicles located in the frontal scalp.

Through a series of biochemical reactions, these enzymes convert testosterone and other androgens into another form, known as dihydrotestosterone (DHT). (See Figure 3-1.)

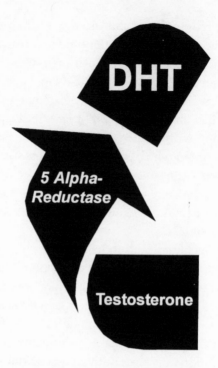

Figure 3-1. Testosterone is the most abundant androgen (male hormone) in women and men. It is converted into DHT by the enzyme, 5 alpha-reductase. DHT is the hormone that triggers androgenetic alopecia.

DHT and Androgenetic Alopecia

DHT is your hair's worst enemy. In a process called *miniaturization*, DHT shrinks hair follicles and causes them to deteriorate over time, triggering hair loss. With miniaturization, the tiny blood vessels nourishing the follicle diminish, cutting off the vital flow of nutrients to the surrounding scalp. Many of the current antibaldness medications on the worldwide market are designed to block the conversion of testosterone into DHT, and some are formulated to stimulate the formation of new blood vessels.

Ironically, one of DHT's normal functions is to promote hair loss! But if your hair follicles have a genetically predetermined sensitivity to DHT, those follicles will shrink and wither.

The enzyme *aromatase*, present in the root of the follicle, plays a protective role against androgenetic alopecia. It converts some testosterone and DHT into estrogen, a female hormone. To a certain extent, estrogen guards the follicles from the effects of androgens. In fact, aromatase is six times more abundant on parts of a woman's scalp than on a man's, which may partly explain why women are less prone to balding than men are.

With androgenetic alopecia, you may lose your hair gradually, but you will never go completely bald. And with proper treatment, hair loss is partially reversible.

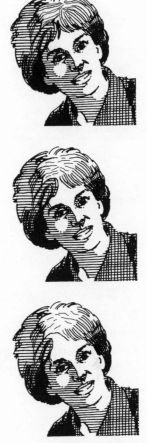

Antiandrogens to the Rescue

The goal of treating androgenetic alopecia is to curtail hormonal activity in the hair follicle, either by blocking the conversion of testosterone to DHT, reversing or stabilizing the miniaturization process, or enhancing the conversion of androgens to estrogens.

A powerful class of drugs, antiandrogens, can mount the required defense and sabotage the activity of androgens such as DHT. In women, these drugs

Figure 3-2. Androgenetic alopecia in women: patterns of hair loss

have been used to treat a broad range of conditions, including symptoms of polycystic ovary disease, hirsutism (excessive hair growth), acne, seborrhea, and hair loss—see Table 3-1 on page 18 for a list of antiandrogens.

There are two classes of antiandrogens: steroidal and nonsteroidal. Steroidal antiandrogens are hormones, whereas nonsteroidal

Table 3-1. Medicines with Antiandrogen Activity

ANTIANDROGENS	5 ALPHA-REDUCTASE INHIBITORS
Cimetidine (Tagamet)	Azelaic Acid (Azelex)
Cyproterone Acetate (Androcur)	Estrogens (Premarin, Estrace)
Flutamide (Eulexin)	Finasteride (Propecia)
Ketoconazole (Nizoral)	
Spironolactone (Aldactone)	

antiandrogens have no hormonal activity. They were developed as potentially safer, less risky alternatives to steroidal antiandrogens.

How Antiandrogens Work

These drugs foil the activity of androgens in one of three ways. Antiandrogens:

- Suppress the production of androgens.
- Inhibit androgen metabolism—that is, antiandrogens prevent the body from handling, or using, androgens, in a normal way.
- Block androgen activity at the cellular level.

This latter action needs further elaboration. An androgen gets hooked—like a key in a lock—to receptors (cellular keyholes) in the cells where it is intended to work. But along comes an antiandrogen, and it changes the lock! Thus, the androgens circulating in the blood can't get in and influence the hair follicles. This is basically how antiandrogens block the cellular activity of androgens.

Types of Antiandrogens

There are many types of antiandrogens, some available only in Europe and Canada. Although they can make hair regrow and slow the progression of hair loss, none are approved by the U.S. Food and Drug Administration (FDA) as hair-loss treatments but are authorized only for the treatment of other medical conditions. Hair regrowth just happens to be one of their side effects.

Even so, many physicians and dermatologists recommend antiandrogens for hair loss, anyway. *It is important to point out that while being treated with antiandrogens, you should not get pregnant. According to current medical literature on antiandrogens, these drugs can potentially feminize a male fetus.*

5 Alpha-Reductase Inhibitors

Another avenue of treatment for androgenetic alopecia is a recently developed class of drugs called *5 alpha-reductase inhibitors*. These drugs block the action of androgens by a different route: They decrease the activity of the enzymes required to convert testosterone into DHT. Table 3-1 on page 18 includes a list of alpha-reductase inhibitors.

In Part 2, you'll learn about the numerous drugs available to treat androgenetic alopecia, including antiandrogens and 5 alpha-reductase inhibitors.

Recognizing and Treating Androgenetic Alopecia

SYMPTOMS
- Diffuse hair thinning
- Hair thinning on the crown
- Increased shedding
- Widening part
- Less hair volume
- Thinner hair shafts
- Increased greasiness of scalp

TREATMENTS
- Minoxidil
- Antiandrogens
- Estrogens
- Retin-A (tretinoin)
- Commercial, nondrug treatments

ALTERNATIVE THERAPIES
- ElectroTrichoGenesis (ETG)
- Diet and nutrition
- Nutritional supplements
- Herbs

HAIR-RESTORATION TECHNIQUES
- Hair transplantation
- Nonsurgical hair systems

TELOGEN EFFLUVIUM
The second most common form of hair loss is *telogen effluvium*, usually triggered by severe physical or emotional stress, but also by other causes. Together, telogen effluvium and androgenetic alopecia account for about 95 percent of all hair-loss cases.

With telogen effluvium, an abnormally high percentage of actively growing hairs abruptly enter telogen, the resting phase of hair growth. The cells in the hair's matrix appear to stop dividing. Consequently, hair begins to fall out. It affects mostly women in their forties, fifties, and sixties. With telogen effluvium, your hair may begin to fall out in clumps, and the shedding may last two to three months, or longer.

There are three types of telogen effluvium: sudden, delayed and chronic.

Sudden Telogen Effluvium
This type of shedding usually begins in response to bodily stress, such as a high fever. Hair loss occurs quite suddenly and rapidly.

Delayed Telogen Effluvium
This form can strike within several months after you undergo extreme physical or psychological stress, such as a severe illness or major surgery. Example: If you have a total hysterectomy, you may experience hair thinning a few months afterward. Accidents

or the death of a parent or child have also been known to trigger this form of telogen effluvium.

If you notice handfuls of hair coming out in your comb or brush during the weeks following the birth of your baby, rest assured that the shedding is fairly common. It, too, is a form of delayed telogen effluvium.

After delivery, your hair may retreat into its resting phase and begin to fall out. But within four to eight months it will start growing again. Some women, however, report that their new hair is not as thick as it was prior to pregnancy. Others find that pregnancy permanently changes their hair color, or relaxes their curls.

Chronic Telogen Effluvium
If the shedding persists for months or years, you may have *chronic telogen effluvium*. Hair is usually lost from the entire scalp. But rest assured: Total baldness is not the end result.

One of the most telling symptoms of chronic telogen effluvium is *trichodynia*, or painful hair. Your hair feels like it is being plucked or pricked by needles. Trichodynia occurs in about 30 percent of all chronic telogen effluvium cases. It's more common in women experiencing depression. In fact, one researcher has noted that depressed women with marital problems are among the most prone to trichodynia. It's not clear, however, why this link exists.

Diagnostically, it can be hard for you or your doctor to tell whether you are suffering from chronic telogen effluvium or androgenetic alopecia. Table 3-2 on page 22 compares the telltale signs of each disease.

Diet and Telogen Effluvium
Insufficient protein in your diet can lead to telogen effluvium. When protein is in short supply, your body tries to conserve as much as possible. One of its defense mechanisms is to shift growing hairs into their resting stage, and those hairs eventually fall out. Eating more protein, however, reverses this type of hair loss.

Table 3-2. Differences Between Chronic Telogen Effluvium
and Androgenetic Alopecia

ANDROGENETIC ALOPECIA	CHRONIC TELOGEN EFFLUVIUM
• Shedding may increase in the fall.	• Shedding occurs at any time throughout the year.
• No event precipitates hair loss.	• Hair loss can be tied to a specific stressful event.
• No trichodynia.	• Trichodynia (hair pain) may exist.
• Weekly hair loss is more gradual and not as extensive in the early stages.	• Weekly hair loss is extensive (100 to 1,000 hairs a week).
• Thinning may be worse on the crown.	• Crown is usually intact, with general thinning over the entire scalp.
• Numerous miniaturized hairs.	• No miniaturized hairs.
• Has a genetic component.	• No genetic component.

SOURCE: Adapted from A. Rebora. 1997. Telogen Effluvium. *Dermatology* 195: 209–12.

Crash dieters and some vegetarians are at risk of losing their hair due to protein deficiencies.

Occasionally, a shortage of iron in your diet will also produce telogen effluvium. Blood tests easily detect low iron levels, and you can correct the condition by taking iron supplements and eating iron-rich foods.

Women who suffer from eating disorders such as anorexia or bulimia often experience telogen effluvium as a result of severe nutritional deficiencies.

Nonchronic Telogen Effluvium
In nonchronic cases, telogen effluvium is reversible and growth returns to normal on its own. No treatment is required, although some physicians may prescribe a mild tranquilizer to calm jangled nerves. Quite often, when patients take antianxiety medication, their hair shedding slows down. This is not a result of the medication but rather a result of their calmer mental state.

SYMPTOMS
- Increased shedding
- Reduced "ponytail" volume
- Normal hair thickness
- Normal scalp surface
- Trichodynia (hair pain)

TREATMENTS
- Corticosteroids such as prednisolone (for chronic telogen effluvium)
- Nioxin, Nisim New Hair Biofactors, or Kevis lotions (for childbirth-related telogen effluvium)
- None, since spontaneous recovery usually occurs.

ALTERNATIVE THERAPIES
- Diet and nutrition
- Nutritional supplements

HAIR-RESTORATION TECHNIQUES
- Nonsurgical hair systems

HAIR-PULLING

A fairly common cause of hair loss is *trichotillomania*, or habitual hair-pulling, a behavior that was identified in 1889 by a French dermatologist. Unlike androgenetic alopecia, telogen effluvium, or other types of hair loss, trichotillomania is not a medical problem but rather a psychological disorder.

The word *trichotillomania* comes from the Greek words for hair, *thrix*; to pull, *tillein*; and for madness, *mania*. Someone with trichotillomania plucks out her hair, strand by strand, in response to inner tension. Stress increases hair pulling, although the behavior also occurs during times of relaxation—while watching television or reading a book, for example. Most sufferers pull out their scalp hair.

Psychiatrists categorize the behavior as an impulse control disorder—a category that includes compulsive gambling and compulsive stealing (kleptomania).

In the fourth edition of the American Psychiatric Association's *Diagnostic and Statistical Manual of Mental Disorders* (DSM), trichotillomania is described formally as:

- Recurrent pulling out of one's hair resulting in noticeable hair loss.
- An increasing sense of tension immediately before pulling out the hair or when attempting to resist the behavior.
- Pleasure, gratification, or relief when pulling out the hair.
- The disturbance is not better accounted for by another mental disorder and is not due to a general medical condition (e.g., a dermatological condition).
- The disturbance causes clinically significant distress in social, occupational, or other important areas of functioning.

Approximately 8 million people in the United States have this condition. Most are adult women. Research indicates that hair-pullers have low self-esteem, suffer from anxiety, experience frequent bouts of depression, and are dissatisfied with their bodies.

Trichotillomania usually begins in childhood and can be successfully treated by psychological counseling and stress management techniques. When trichotillomania is suspected, a dermatologist may take a skin biopsy to look for scalp hemorrhaging and empty hair follicles.

Psychiatrists also treat trichotillomania, often by advising patients to wear gloves or smear petroleum jelly on their hands. These practices blunt the touch sensation and keep the sufferer from pulling out her hair.

Hair usually grows back, although repeated pulling over many years may permanently destroy hair follicles. There is a national organization for people with trichotillomania that can provide information on support groups, as well as additional resources; see Appendix B on page 220 for information.

SYMPTOMS
- One or a few well-defined areas of hair loss
- Abnormal redness of the scalp around the follicles
- Scalp hemorrhaging
- Empty hair follicles

TREATMENT
- Behavioral counseling
- Stress resolution
- Clomipramine (Anafranil), a drug made by Novartis and used to treat obsessive-compulsive disorder

HAIR-RESTORATION TECHNIQUES
- Nonsurgical hair systems

ALOPECIA AREATA
It starts with a tiny bald spot on your head, no bigger than the tip of a felt marker. Within months, it spreads to the size of a penny, then a quarter. Before long, you have only sprigs of hair sticking out from an otherwise hairless scalp.

You're suffering from alopecia areata, a disease that strikes adults and children randomly—even those in very good health. More than 2 million Americans of all ages have it, and it affects men and women alike.

No one knows what causes alopecia areata, although it is thought to be an autoimmune disorder in which the body mistakenly attacks the hair follicles. Inflammation of the follicles and surrounding hair

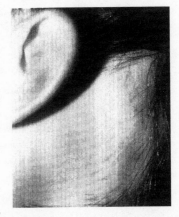

Figure 3.3. Alopecia areata

structures sets in. This reaction causes the hair follicles to retreat into the deeper layers of skin. Shut off from a nutrient supply, the follicles starve, begin shedding hair, and enter a dormant period.

Hair loss due to alopecia areata can occur very rapidly, or slowly, or at irregular intervals. About 25 percent of people with alopecia areata have a family history of the disease. Stress can also trigger alopecia areata, as can exposure to industrial chemicals.

And it can get worse—with hair loss over the entire body—before it gets better. The severest forms of the disease are *alopecia totalis*, hair loss on 100 percent of your scalp; and *alopecia universalis*, hair loss over the whole body.

Treating Alopecia Areata

There's no cure for alopecia areata, but there are numerous treatments that are quite effective. And in many cases, some or all of your hair grows back on its own, whether or not you undergo treatment. If your hair loss is patchy, your hair will probably come back. But if you've been losing your hair for five years or more, your chances are not as good. Unfortunately, there is a high relapse rate for alopecia areata, even after treatment.

Generally, treatment has three goals: to trigger hair growth, to halt the spread of the disease, and to reduce the time intervals between hair shedding and normal hair growth.

Treatment for alopecia depends on two main variables: your age and the extent of your hair loss. Children under ten are usually treated with minoxidil, with or without a topical corticosteroid, or a tarlike ointment called anthralin.

Patients age ten or older receive more aggressive treatment. Your dermatologist will first examine your scalp to pinpoint how much hair you've lost. If less than 50 percent of your hair is gone, your treatment will likely involve:

- Intralesional injections of corticosteroids or a twice-daily application of a 5 percent minoxidil solution (see pages 62–71)

- A high-potency topical corticosteroid cream (see page 48)

If more than 50 percent of your hair is gone, your dermatologist may recommend:

- Treatment with a topical contact sensitizer (see page 77)
- Intralesional injections of corticosteroids in patchy areas that are resistant to topical contact agents (see page 50)
- A 5 percent minoxidil solution applied twice a day, with or without high-potency topical corticosteroids; six months of anthralin therapy; or, possibly, ultraviolet light therapy, otherwise known as PUVA. These are usually tried if therapy with topical contact agents fails.

Because severe alopecia areata is a devastating disease psychologically, you may want to consider joining a support group. The National Alopecia Areata Foundation (NAAF) can help you locate a group in your area, plus supply you with helpful information about the disease, including brochures, newsletters, research updates, and sources for wigs and hairpieces. For information on how to contact the NAAF, see Appendix B (page 223).

Your dermatologist will likely continue treatment until your disease enters remission. Keep in mind, too, that your hair may start regrowing again spontaneously, with or without treatment.

Other Options

Drugs to treat alopecia areata often produce unbearable side effects, and there is the real possibility that they may do nothing for you at all. If you go completely bald, you may have to face a "moment of truth": that your chances of reversing the condition are quite slim. It is at this point that many women give up on drugs and other treatments—but not on themselves. They accept their baldness and get on with their lives.

For appearance's sake, they often decide to wear wigs—well-crafted, well-designed wigs that are indistinguishable from real hair. This is an option chosen by thousands of women with alopecia areata—one with the potential to make you feel better about yourself and the way you look. (For more information on wigs and other types of hair systems, see pages 202–210, as well as Appendix B on page 220.)

Recognizing and Treating Alopecia Areata

SYMPTOMS
- Sudden, patchy hair loss on the scalp
- Quarter-sized, round, smooth bald spots on the scalp and other hair-bearing portions of the body
- General thinning of scalp hair
- Shedding
- The presence of *exclamation point hairs* (short hairs that taper as they approach the scalp surface)
- Loss of scalp, eyebrow, and eyelash hair
- Complete loss of hair over the entire body

TREATMENTS
- Corticosteroids
- Topical contact sensitizers
- Anthralin
- Retin-A (tretinoin)
- Topical minoxidil
- Zinc
- PUVA treatment
- Immunosuppressive drugs
- Commercial, nondrug treatments

ALTERNATIVE THERAPIES
- Diet and nutrition
- Nutritional supplements
- Herbs

HAIR-RESTORATION TECHNIQUES
- Nonsurgical hair systems

DRUG- AND SUPPLEMENT-INDUCED HAIR LOSS

While there are many promising drugs that promote hair growth, there are many more that cause hair to thin or fall out altogether. And rarely do doctors tell you that baldness is a potential side effect of a drug they prescribe. You may have to dig up this information for yourself, or have your doctor look up the side effects in the *Physicians' Desk Reference* for you.

Chemotherapy and Hair Loss

Hair loss is a well-known side effect of many cancer chemotherapy drugs. These medications attack the fast-dividing hair cells of the matrix, and hair is lost from 90 percent or more of the scalp. Within a few weeks after cancer therapy ends, however, hair grows back. Even so, long-term exposure to chemotherapeutic drugs may cause scarring alopecia. Hair loss caused by chemotherapy and other drugs is known as *anagen effluvium*.

Prescription Drugs

Many common prescription drugs thin out hair, too. These include: antidepressants, pain medications, blood thinners, high blood pressure medications, and some cholesterol-lowering drugs. In certain cases, birth control pills also cause hair loss. Case in point: If you have an inherited tendency toward hair loss *and* you take birth control pills, the pills may cause your hair to fall out. In this instance, talk to your doctor about switching to a different pill. Taking an estrogen-dominant pill, for example, may help against further fallout.

Fortunately, drug-induced hair loss is temporary. For a list of drugs that may cause hair loss, see Table 3-3 on page 30.

Dietary Supplements

Certain dietary supplements can be culprits in hair loss. For example, megadoses of vitamin A (in excess of 50,000 international units daily) can promote hair loss. So can DHEA, a popular supplement thought to slow down the aging process. DHEA,

Table 3-3. Drugs That May Cause Hair Loss

THERAPEUTIC CLASS	NAME
Antibiotics	Benzimidazoles gentamicin (Garamycin) nitrofurantoin (Macrodantin) Paraminosalicylates
Anticoagulants	heparin warfarin (Coumadin)
Cardiovascular drugs	amiodarone (Cordarone) captopril enalapril (Vaseretic, Vasotec) methyldopa (Aldomet) nadolol propranolol (Inderal, Inderide)
Chemotherapeutic drugs	Various—check with your physician
Endocrine drugs	bromocriptine (Parlodel) clomiphene citrate (Clomid) danazol (Danocrine)
Immune system drugs	immunoglobulin IV interferon alpha interferon gamma
Lipid-lowering drugs	clofibrate (Atromid-S) fenofibrate (Tricor)
Pain relievers/anti-inflammatories	ibuprofen (Advil, Motrin) indomethacin (Indocin) naproxen (Anaprox, Naprosyn)
Retinoids	isotretinoin (Accutane)
Rheumatic disease drugs	allopurinol (Zyloprim) antimalarials colchicine (ColBENEMID) penicillamine (Cuprimine)

SOURCE: Adapted from: J. Graedon and T. Graedon. 1989. Common drugs cause hair loss. *Medical SelfCare*, November-December, 23; and J. J. Dominique, M. D. Van Neste, and D. H. Rushton. 1997. Hair problems in women. *Clinics in Dermatology*, 15: 113–25.

however, is converted into DHT and thus contributes to hair loss, particularly in certain sensitive individuals. Further, there is insufficient proof that DHEA is beneficial and that it may produce other side effects such as confusion, headaches, drowsiness, liver damage, as well as breast cancer.

A few herbs have been associated with hair loss, too. One of these is astralagus, a popular immune-boosting herb. It contains a natural chemical called *selenocystathionine*, known to cause hair loss. Hair is very high in the mineral sulfur and sulfur-containing proteins; selenocystathionine interferes with the metabolism of sulfur.

With any type of dietary supplement, including herbal formulations, read the label for its list of ingredients. If you're experiencing hair loss or thinning, stop taking the supplement in question and discuss the matter with your physician.

AGE-RELATED HAIR LOSS

It's inevitable: We all lose hair as we age. Typically, you'll notice a very gradual, diffuse thinning of your scalp hair, starting at about age fifty. Unlike other forms of hair loss, there's usually no noticeable shedding, just a gradual thinning out. If your hair loss is severe in the years following menopause, particularly on the frontal scalp, then you're probably suffering from androgenetic alopecia as well. There's no specific treatment for age-related hair loss. However, certain supportive treatments such as proper diet and supplementation may help minimize it.

Recognizing and Treating Age-Related Hair Loss

SYMPTOMS
- Gradual, diffuse thinning of scalp hair

ALTERNATIVE THERAPIES
- Diet and nutrition
- Nutritional supplements
- Herbs

HAIR-RESTORATION TECHNIQUES
- Hair transplantation
- Nonsurgical hair systems

DISEASE-RELATED HAIR LOSS
There are a number of diseases that will produce hair loss. When the disease is cured, however, hair loss will usually reverse itself. Diseases that commonly cause hair loss are discussed below.

Syphilitic Alopecia

If you're losing your hair for no apparent reason and other causes have been ruled out, your physician may examine you for syphilis, a three-stage bacterial disease transmitted by sexual contact or through infected blood.

Up to 20 percent of patients with syphilis begin to go bald. The symptoms of syphilitic alopecia include either patchy or diffuse hair loss on the scalp or other parts of the body, or a combination of patchy and diffuse thinning. The patches of baldness give the scalp a moth-eaten appearance. Hair loss may be rapid or slow, and you may have pimplelike sores on your scalp.

A diagnosis of syphilis can be confirmed by blood tests. If caught early and treated appropriately, syphilis can be completely cured. If not treated, the disease leads to death.

Syphilis is treated with antibiotics, and hair growth returns to normal after the disease is cured.

Recognizing and Treating Syphilitic Alopecia

SYMPTOMS
- Patchy hair loss
- Diffuse thinning
- The presence of pimplelike sores on the scalp

TREATMENT
- Antibiotics

Thyroid Disease

Thyroid disease can lead to hair loss. *Hyperthyroidism* occurs when the thyroid gland overproduces thyroid hormone—a condition that may cause hair to fall out. An underactive thyroid leads to *hypothyroidism*, and one of its symptoms is also hair loss. In both diseases, hair loss can be reversed with proper medication. Hair starts growing a few months after thyroid hormone levels have normalized.

Bacterial Infections

A fairly common type of disease-related hair loss is bacterial infection. One of these is *folliculitis*, an infection of the hair follicles. Small, pus-filled pimples form around the hair follicles, and hair may thin out. Another type of bacterial infection is *pyoderma*, which makes the skin red and scaly. The presence of bacterial infections can be confirmed by culture tests. Bacterial infections can be treated topically or by oral medications, depending on the severity of the disease.

Fungal Infections

Although rare in adults, fungal infections such as ringworm often lead to hair loss. The presence of a fungal infection can be confirmed by a culture. Hair loss caused by ringworm is treated with an antifungal drug called griseofulvin (Gris-PEG, Grisactin, or Fulvicin- P/G), and occasionally with oral steroids if inflammation is present.

Seborrhea and Psoriasis

Skin disorders such as seborrhea and psoriasis can lead to hair loss also. Seborrhea occurs when the sebaceous glands become overactive, resulting in excessive production of sebum. Treatment often involves the use of medicated shampoos and antiandrogen drugs.

Affecting approximately 3 million Americans, psoriasis is a genetic disease in which the life cycle of skin cells fast-forward abnormally, and the result is skin eruptions and scaling. Psoriasis typically affects the elbows, knees, trunk, and scalp. Treatment involves medications and phototherapy (exposure of the skin to ultraviolet light).

SCARRING ALOPECIA

Scarring alopecia is a form of baldness caused by chemical or physical burns to the scalp, as well as by various scalp infections and diseases. These can include skin tumors, *erythematosis discoid lupus* (an immune system disorder that affects the skin), *scleroderma* (a thickening of the skin), and *lichen planus* (a rare but recurrent skin rash). Fungal infections can also cause scarring alopecia. Medically, scarring alopecia is sometimes referred to as *cicatricial alopecia*.

In scarring alopecia, the scarred areas appear pale, glazy, and smooth. Unlike other types of hair loss, hairs in their growing (anagen) phase are easily plucked out. The hair follicles are damaged, and the resulting baldness is usually irreversible. However, some dermatologists take an aggressive approach to treatment, particularly where a disease such as lupus is involved, to arrest the scarring process. Treatment often includes topical, oral, and injectable steroids; retinoids such as Retin-A; or antibiotic treatments such as shampoos or topical treatments. Antimalarial agents such as hydroxychloroquine have also been used to treat scarring alopecia.

COSMETICALLY INDUCED HAIR LOSS

A form of hair loss that may be categorized as either scarring or nonscarring alopecia is cosmetically induced hair loss. It is caused by certain hairstyles and the use of chemicals.

Hairstyles

Wearing tight hairstyles such as pigtails, ponytails, cornrows, or using tight rollers can pull on your hair, causing hair to fall out.

This type of hair loss is called *traction alopecia*. In many cases, it will scar your scalp. But provided there is no scarring, your hair will grow back normally after you stop the pulling.

Another hairstyle that can lead to hair loss is the bun, or chignon. Regularly wearing your hair in a tight bun or ponytail can cause baldness at the hairline—a condition some dermatologists have dubbed *chignon alopecia*.

Hair Relaxers and Hot Combs

African-American women have to be especially careful in their beauty regimens. Styling techniques such as cornrowing, hair relaxers, and hot combs can unknowingly contribute to hair and scalp disease, according to Dr. Gary J. Brauner, a dermatologist who has extensively studied and published scientific research related to skin diseases in African Americans.

"The frequent use of chemical hair relaxers to straighten the waves of African-American hair weakens the hair, even when done properly," he said. "And if hair relaxers are combined with tight hair rolling, it almost always leads to hair loss."

Some hair relaxers have been known to cause scalp irritation and hair discoloration. In 1994, the FDA issued a warning for one such product after consumers complained that it caused their hair to fall out or turn green. Consequently, the manufacturer stopped all sales and shipments of the product.

An alternate method of relaxing hair, the hot comb, uses a heated metal comb and petroleum jelly or oil. This method usually leads to progressive, often irreversible hair loss, beginning at the crown and spreading across the entire head.

Dyes, Bleaches, and Permanent Waves

In addition, chemical treatments such as dyes, bleaches, or permanent waves, if applied incorrectly, can weaken the hair and cause breakage. In extreme cases, hair can even fall out. Further, an allergic reaction to hair dye can also cause hair loss.

Wilma F. Bergfeld, M.D., F.A.C.P.
1992 President of the American Academy of Dermatology
Head of Dermatology, Clinical Research and Dermatopathology at the Cleveland Clinic

Dr. Bergfeld specializes in treating hair loss, androgenetic alopecia, and androgen excess. For women experiencing androgenetic alopecia, she advises the following steps:

"First, a dermatologist should take a good history of hair loss events, both acute and chronic. In addition, a personal medical history, drug history, menstrual period history, and family history are important. Many factors induce hair loss and shedding, and some even mimic or exaggerate genetic hair loss. Therefore, identification of all the triggers or causes of hair loss can reduce or minimize the cosmetic problem.

"The next step is to have the dermatologist examine the scalp and body, skin and hair distribution, and hair type and density. The presence of scalp skin disease such as seborrheic dermatitis frequently accompanies androgenetic alopecia and is a symptom of androgen excess."

After medical tests and scalp examinations have been performed, Dr. Bergfeld recommends the following course of treatment:

1. Antiseborrheic shampoo, one to three times a week; anti-inflammatory lotions such as hydrocortisone; and nutritional advice and supplements. (See Dr. Bergfeld's comments on nutrition therapy on page 135.)

2. Two percent topical minoxidil, applied twice a day for a year; and if needed, 5 percent topical minoxidil twice a day. It takes four to twelve months to see any appreciable growth. Shedding is reduced in two to four months. In rare cases, a patient will experience increased shedding with minoxidil, but this generally resolves and hair begins to grow in about four months. With the 5 percent minoxidil, women can experience increased facial hair

and, in rare cases, increased body hair (known technically as hirsutism). This growth is dose-dependent. It will disappear when the drug is stopped, or will lessen if you use a reduced amount or use it less frequently.

"If hair growth plateaus at one year, increase the strength or frequency of application," she adds. "Minoxidil is sold as an over-the-counter medication, at 2 percent and 5 percent concentrations. Only the 2 percent formulation is generic.

"Confusion has developed over which products are meant solely for women, as opposed to those for men. The women's product is packaged in pink; the men's product in blue. The bottom line is that they work the same in both sexes. Minoxidil is the first FDA-approved drug for hair growth, and is available as Rogaine (2 percent) and Extra Strength Rogaine For Men (5 percent)."

Dr. Bergfeld adds that there are other helpful therapies for women that are not yet approved by the FDA. "The use of hormones, in the form of birth control pills and hormone replacement therapy (HRT), is frequently helpful. So is spironolactone (Aldactone), an androgen blocker. Clinical studies and case reports alone and in combination with birth control pills or hormone replacement therapy demonstrate decreased shedding and increased hair growth. Large clinical trials have not been done, however.

"The discovery of a thyroid disorder and subsequent treatment improves hair growth. The correction of minor to severe anemias with an over-the-counter iron supplements is also helpful in reducing shedding and initiating regrowth."

FOUR

Pinpointing the Cause of Your Hair Loss

I F YOU NOTICE unusual hair loss, see your doctor (preferably a dermatologist) as soon as you can. Hair loss and thinning can lead to fear, anxiety, and depression—all of which can seriously affect physical health. Proper treatment can help reverse hair loss and, in doing so, erase much of the psychological discomfort you are experiencing.

Assist Your Physician in Making a More Accurate Diagnosis

You can help your doctor or dermatologist arrive at a more accurate diagnosis. Prior to your appointment, scribble down the facts behind your hair loss and general health by answering these questions:

- How long have you been losing your hair?
- When did the hair loss start?
- Is your hair coming out by the roots or breaking off?
- Have you had any recent illnesses or surgery?
- Do you have a family history of baldness?
- Are you taking any medications or supplements?
- What is your normal diet?
- Have you experienced sudden, unexplained weight loss?

- Have you had a recent pregnancy, hysterectomy, or experienced any menstrual irregularities?
- What kind of hair care products do you use, including shampoos, conditioners, chemicals (rinses, bleaches, straighteners, or permanents)?
- What do you use to style your hair (electric rollers, dryers, hot curlers, regular rollers, teasing, or use of rubber bands)?

In addition, bring in a photograph of yourself taken a few years earlier when you had more hair, or a handful of hair that has recently fallen out.

All of this information will help your physician or dermatologist take a detailed medical history, which is usually the first step in making an accurate diagnosis. Your medical history will help your doctor sort out whether your problem is a physiological response to stress, a reaction to a drug or supplement, a side effect of an illness, an inherited tendency, or a cosmetically induced problem.

Diagnostic Tests

Quite probably, your doctor will conduct and order some specific tests. These may include:

SCALP EXAMINATION

Your dermatologist will examine your scalp to determine patterns of hair thinning. Diffuse thinning, for example, is often a sign of androgenetic alopecia.

Alopecia areata is characterized by various patterns of hair loss. You may have a snakelike path of hair loss around the back and sides of your scalp; patches of hair loss in a grid formation all over your scalp; a triangular patch of hair loss; or diffuse thinning all over your scalp. The appearance of diffuse thinning often makes it hard to distinguish alopecia areata from androgenetic alopecia.

In addition, a scalp examination can reveal whether there is inflammation or signs of a fungal or bacterial infection. If an infection is suspected, a culture will be taken.

HAIR-PULL TEST

With a hair-pull test, your dermatologist will gently tug on about eight to ten of your hairs to see how many come out. Losing two hairs is normal; the loss of four or more is not.

A hair-pull test helps a dermatologist diagnose or rule out alopecia areata and other forms of baldness. To check for alopecia areata, for example, your dermatologist will grasp and lightly pull on a group of hairs near patchy areas. If six or more hairs are easily removed, the disease is active, and you may lose more hair. But if hair is not easily pulled out around those patches, you probably won't lose any more hair. Furthermore, if hair is easily plucked out over your entire scalp, you may be in danger of losing all your scalp hair to alopecia areata.

MICROSCOPIC EVALUATION

Your dermatologist may also examine the plucked hairs and roots under a microscope, count the number of anagen and telogen hairs, and contrast that number to a normal count. An abnormal number of telogen hairs often helps confirm or rule out the diagnosis of telogen effluvium.

Under the microscope, the root of an anagen hair will appear pigmented; the root of a telogen hair will not. If 50 percent or more hairs are in the telogen phase, then your excessive shedding may be due to telogen effluvium.

SCALP BIOPSY

A scalp biopsy may be required as well. It helps exclude other causes of hair loss.

Your dermatologist will trim some hair in the area of the biopsy specimen and inject the area with a local anesthetic. Using a special tool, he or she will remove a tiny, 4- to 5-millimeter section of your scalp, then sew up the opening. A topical antibiotic will be applied, and you can gently shampoo your hair the next day. The biopsy is examined under a microscope.

A scalp biopsy is the most accurate way to diagnose alopecia areata. Scalp tissue is examined to detect abnormal immune activity, stunted growth, and inflammation. The results of the biopsy help determine the appropriate therapy.

OTHER TESTS

Additional tests may be ordered. These include:

- Thyroid tests to detect abnormal thyroid functioning.
- Blood tests to exclude low iron or ferritin levels. (Ferritin is an iron-containing protein synthesized in the liver and found in the blood.) A blood test can also screen for shortages in other nutrients, or determine whether you have syphilis.
- Laboratory screening tests for elevated androgens, or a hormonal imbalance. Either could be a sign that hair loss is due to androgenetic alopecia.

PART 2

Mane Medications From A to Z

Antibaldness Medications

A s of 1999, the only medicines that have been officially approved by the Food and Drug Administration to treat hair loss are minoxidil, better known by one of its trade names, Rogaine; and finasteride, or Propecia. Finasteride, however, is not recommended for women because of its numerous health risks, including birth defects. Minoxidil, better known as Rogaine, is available as both an over-the-counter drug (the 2 percent version) and as a prescription medication (the 5 percent version).

There are many other drugs that effectively fight baldness, but they are not yet officially approved to do so. Nonetheless, many dermatologists are successfully using them to treat hair loss in women. These drugs are described in this section.

All the antibaldness medications listed here are classified as drugs. As a handy reference, they are listed alphabetically.

Anthralin (Micanol, Drithocreme, Drithro-Scalp)
Used to treat alopecia areata, anthralin is a tarlike ointment applied to the scalp. Normally, it is prescribed to fight the skin disease psoriasis. Micanol is manufacturered by Bioglan; Drithocreme and Drithro-Scalp by Dermik.

HOW DOES IT WORK?
Anthralin counteracts cell division and prevents the overproduction of skin cells covering the scalp.

HOW IS IT USED?
Anthralin is applied either in a high concentration for a short period of time (up to one hour) on alternating days, or in lower

concentrations daily, usually overnight. Your dermatologist will instruct you to shampoo the medication off at the end of the prescribed time period.

WHEN WILL I SEE RESULTS?

When the treatment works, some new hair growth appears within two to three months. But it may take two years or longer to obtain meaningful hair growth.

Even so, results from using anthralin are mixed. In a study conducted at the University of Illinois in 1987, investigators found that the medication regrew hair in seventeen (25 percent) out of sixty-eight patients suffering from alopecia areata. It took roughly twenty-three weeks of use before results were seen.

What this study hints at is that anthralin may work as a hair restorer for some people with alopecia areata. Thus, it may be worth a try.

ARE THERE SIDE EFFECTS?

Side effects are rare, but may include skin irritation, according to the *Physicians' Desk Reference*. Withholding treatment for a few days will heal this condition.

If you use anthralin, wash your hands after each application to keep from getting it in your eyes.

Azelaic Acid (Azelex)

Available as a 20 percent cream, azelaic acid is a topical medication normally used to treat acne. It may also be helpful in treating androgenetic alopecia. Azelex is made by Allergan.

Azelaic acid is a naturally occurring compound found in whole grain cereals and some animal products. In addition, our bodies can make azelaic acid from a fatty acid called oleic acid.

HOW DOES IT WORK?

Studies on azelaic acid conducted in the eighties revealed that it is also a powerful inhibitor of the 5 alpha-reductase enzymes, which are required to convert testosterone into DHT. When combined with zinc and vitamin B$_6$, azelaic acid can block the action of these enzymes by 90 percent. This finding has led researchers to speculate that the medication might be effective against androgenetic alopecia. However, no studies have yet investigated azelaic acid as an antibaldness remedy, so it is not clear how much to use, or what the outcome might be.

Azelaic acid is found in a prescription hair-loss remedy known as Xandrox, which also contains minoxidil and other healing ingredients. Refer to the section below for more information on Xandrox.

HOW IS IT USED?

The product comes in tubes with instructions to massage the affected areas twice a day—in the morning and evening. When azelaic acid is part of a hair-loss remedy such as Xandrox, it is applied topically to the scalp.

ARE THERE SIDE EFFECTS?

Generally, azelaic acid has very few side effects. In some cases, side effects may include rashes, skin inflammation, and a slight loss of skin color, according to the *Physicians' Desk Reference*.

Cimetidine (Tagamet)

You know cimetidine, marketed as Tagamet by SmithKline Beecham, as the pill you pop for acid indigestion, heartburn, or ulcers. Available as an over-the-counter medication, it soothes these conditions and is a very effective drug in that regard. Cimetidine has also been studied as a potential remedy against androgenetic alopecia.

HOW DOES IT WORK?

When taken in multiple daily doses, cimetidine acts like an antiandrogen. It prevents androgens from latching on to their cellular receptors. In that role, cimetidine helps activate hair regrowth.

HOW IS IT USED?

It's not clear yet what the most effective dosage might be, or whether cimetidine should even be used to treat hair loss. But in a 1987 study, ten women with moderate to severe androgenetic alopecia took 300 milligrams of cimetidine orally five times day. They stayed on the drug for an average of five months. Seven patients showed good to excellent regrowth of their hair, and no major side effects were reported.

The dosage used in this study was only slightly higher than what is normally prescribed for ulcer patients. In other words, the amount that sparks hair regrowth is not a megadose.

While this is a fascinating study, more research into the antibalding effects of cimetidine is needed. Because it is not approved for treating baldness, do not take cimetidine for hair loss unless you are under medical supervision.

ARE THERE SIDE EFFECTS?

When cimetidine is taken in normal doses to treat heartburn and ulcers, side effects are rare but not unknown. According to the *Physicians' Desk Reference*, some side effects include agitation, anxiety, breast development in males, depression, headache, mental confusion, and sleepiness.

NOTE: According to the *Physicians' Desk Reference*, before taking cimetidine, check with your doctor if:
- You have kidney or liver disease.
- You are allergic to the drug.
- You are pregnant, plan to become pregnant, or are nursing. (Cimetidine makes its way to breast milk.)
- You are taking other prescription or nonprescription drugs.

Corticosteroids

If you are diagnosed with alopecia areata, your dermatologist will probably prescribe a medicine known as a *corticosteroid*.

In the body, corticosteroids are a group of steroid hormones secreted by the adrenal cortex, one of the adrenal glands. These hormones help the body resist stress caused by injury, illness, mental strain, severe exertion, and allergies. Without the adrenal cortex and its secretion of corticosteroids, your body would buckle under the potentially fatal effects of stress.

The first corticosteroid ever developed was cortisone, originally made from ox bile and later from plant steroids in soybeans and Mexican yams. When introduced more than fifty years ago, cortisone was considered a miracle drug. People crippled with painful, debilitating arthritis could walk again, patients with asthma and allergies could breathe normally, and even those suffering from leukemia and other malignancies went into temporary remission. But amid all the hope, it was soon learned that when the treatment stopped, the symptoms returned, often with severe side effects.

Today, newer, synthetic versions of cortisone—collectively called corticosteroids—have been developed. As medicine, synthetic corticosteroids are a class of powerful drugs used to treat various forms of inflammation and alleviate symptoms in a variety of disorders, including rheumatoid arthritis, severe asthma, and prevention of organ rejection from transplants.

Some of the more common corticosteroids are hydrocortisone, triamcinolone acetonide, prednisone, and prednisolone.

HOW DO CORTICOSTEROIDS WORK?
These drugs work by mimicking the actions of the natural hormones produced in the adrenal glands. The FDA has approved various versions of cortisone for treating a range of ailments but requires comprehensive labeling to make sure physicians understand—and communicate to patients—their risks and benefits.

HOW IS IT USED?
Topical Therapy. Topically applied corticosteroid creams are the mildest form of treatment and usually tried first for treating

alopecia areata. Creams work best if you've had alopecia areata for a short time. According to medical research, it may take about three months for this treatment to produce any meaningful hair growth.

Brands used by dermatologists include Diprosone (a 0.5 percent betamethesone cream), Synalar (0.25 percent fluocinolone acetonide), and Kenalog (triamcinolone acetonide).

But often, alopecia areata doesn't respond to these creams. To increase their effectiveness, physicians often prescribe them in conjunction with injectable and oral corticosteroids (see below).

Many dermatologists with experience in treating alopecia areata believe that topical medications should be applied to the entire scalp, not just to the patchy areas. Full scalp coverage maximizes the potential for cosmetic hair growth.

WHEN WILL I SEE RESULTS?

Meaningful hair growth may take a year or more to achieve. A maintenance treatment program is important, too, since it can help preserve the cosmetic growth already obtained.

According to the *Physicians' Desk Reference*, side effects are rare, although the prescription creams may cause burning, itching, and irritation of the scalp. The use of over-the-counter preparations of topical hydrocortisone rarely produces any serious side effects.

Injections. Mild, patchy cases of alopecia areata may respond well to injections of corticosteroids. In fact, this treatment works best when less than 50 percent of your scalp is affected by the disease.

One of the most-often-used agents is injectable triamcinolone acetonide, injected into the affected site around the follicles. Called an "intralesional injection," this treatment is typically given every four to six weeks.

Hair may start regrowing within two to eight weeks after treatment has begun. If you don't respond after six months, the shots should be stopped. Side effects are rare, but may include weight gain and reddening and rounding of the face and neck. You may also experience pain around the injection site.

Oral Therapy. More severe cases of alopecia areata require oral corticosteroids taken as tablets. The drug prednisone is often prescribed, although it is often considered a last resort. Oral therapy is the most potent form of treatment.

For alopecia areata affecting more than 50 percent of the scalp, an initial treatment regimen of 40 to 60 milligrams of oral prednisone taken daily can stop the sometimes rapid progression of the disease, according to medical research. Some dermatologists may suggest much higher doses. Dosages of prednisone are usually tapered down by 5 milligrams a week to maintain any hair regrowth and avoid problems associated with long-term use. Oral therapy is sometimes used in conjunction with injections.

Prednisolone is another corticosteroid that has been successfully used to treat serious alopecia areata. A 1996 study found that the drug was helpful in treating patients with widespread alopecia areata (baldness over 40 percent of the scalp).

Twenty-seven patients (twenty-one with alopecia areata, five with alopecia universalis, and one with alopecia totalis) were given 300-milligram doses of prednisolone at four-week intervals for a minimum of four doses, or until cosmetically acceptable hair regrowth appeared. A 1,000-milligram dose of prednisolone was administered to eight patients in the same manner. Five of these patients had alopecia totalis; the other three had alopecia areata but had not previously responded to the 300-milligram dose regimen.

After an average of four months, fourteen patients (thirteen with alopecia areata and one with alopecia totalis) taking the 300-milligram doses showed complete or cosmetically acceptable hair growth.

Three patients taking the higher dose had cosmetically acceptable hair growth after six to nine months. One of the patients suffered from alopecia totalis, one from alopecia universalis, and the other from alopecia areata. The researchers concluded that monthly treatment with oral doses of 300 milligrams of prednisolone is effective.

Oral corticosteroids should be used with great caution, however, because the potential for side effects is high. According to the *Physicians' Desk Reference*, psychological side effects include mood changes, psychotic behavior, severe depression, and insomnia. Physical side effects include eye problems (such as cataracts or glaucoma), bone fractures, muscle weakness, poor wound healing, ulcers, weight gain, and skin problems. Prolonged use of corticosteroids can disrupt the normal activity of the adrenal cortex, a part of the adrenal glands that secretes various hormones.

Many physicians believe that early, vigorous treatment of patchy alopecia areata with corticosteroids can prevent the disease from progressing to more untreatable, cosmetically disfiguring forms.

When considering treatment with corticosteroids, be sure to thoroughly discuss the pros and cons with your physician.

NOTE: According to the *Physicians' Desk Reference*, do not use prescription corticosteroids if:

- You have ever had an allergic reaction to any of these drugs.
- You suffer from any disease or infection.
- You are pregnant or planning to become pregnant.
- You have high blood pressure.
- You are under eighteen years of age, unless closely monitored by a physician. Use of corticosteroids by children can stunt growth.

Cyproterone Acetate (Androcur)

Cyproterone acetate (CPA) was one of the first steroidal antiandrogens ever used to treat hair loss. Sold as Androcur, it is available only in Europe and Canada.

HOW DOES IT WORK?

Taken orally, CPA is a synthetic steroid that obstructs the activity of androgens by preventing them from attaching to receptors in the cells of the skin and hair follicles. It also reduces the activity of the ovaries, so that much smaller amounts of androgens are produced.

CPA has been well tested, with results showing minimal to moderate hair growth in women. Most often, it is used in combination with an estrogen (usually ethinyl estradiol). This combination helps reduce levels of testosterone in the body.

According to scientific consensus, one of the most effective regimens is 50 milligrams daily of CPA from day five to day fifteen of the menstrual cycle, along with ethinyl estradiol (30 micrograms daily) from day five to day twenty-four of the cycle. After three years, the dosage of CPA is reduced to 25 milligrams for ten days of the menstrual cycle. This treatment regimen stopped balding in every woman who used it, and increased hair regrowth up to 30 percent in some.

CPA is often prescribed in conjunction with an estrogen-containing birth control pill called Diane-35, available in Europe and Canada. Diane-35 contains 2 milligrams of CPA and 50 micrograms of ethinyl estradiol. It is a low-dose contraceptive that was introduced in the late 1970s as an alternative to other birth control pills. In one study, CPA and Diane-35 improved hair loss in 45 percent of the women who used both agents.

This combination also increases the growth phase of hair, shortens its resting phase, thickens hair fibers, and reduces scalp greasiness.

WHEN WILL I SEE RESULTS?

It may take six months or longer to see these improvements.

ARE THERE SIDE EFFECTS?

In the many studies conducted on CPA, few side effects have been reported. However, some women may experience fatigue, weight gain, irregular uterine bleeding, breast tenderness, or headaches. These side effects are improved when CPA is taken in conjunction with estrogen.

In addition, CPA therapy depletes the body of vitamin B_{12}, required for a healthy nervous system, according to medical studies of the drug. A deficiency is serious, potentially causing irreversible nerve damage. Numbness or tingling in the arms or legs, mental depression, memory loss, weakness, and uncoordination are among the warnings of nerve impairment from a vitamin B_{12} deficiency. Women being treated with CPA and estrogen can prevent a deficiency by taking a daily supplement of vitamin B_{12} in prescribed doses.

Antiandrogen therapy for hair loss works best when the body is well stocked with the mineral iron. Your physician can determine if your iron levels are healthy by giving you a blood test. If you are running low on iron, you may have to take iron supplements. For more information on vitamin B_{12} and iron, see Chapters Nine and Ten.

Leading dermatologists feel that CPA is unlikely to be available in the United States in the near future. You should discuss with your dermatologist whether you can import it for personal use under his or her medical care.

Estrogen

Estrogen is the collective name for a trio of female hormones: estradiol, secreted from the ovaries during reproductive years; estriol, produced by the placenta during pregnancy; and estrone, secreted by the ovaries and adrenal glands and found in women after menopause.

These naturally occurring estrogens are responsible for developing the female sex characteristics, regulating menstrual cycles, and maintaining normal cholesterol levels.

As you approach menopause, your natural level of estrogens falls off. Around this time you may notice that your hair has started to thin. One possible explanation is that reduced levels of estrogens shorten the anagen phase of hair growth. When estrogen is in short supply, your natural protection against hair loss is gone. Hair loss following childbirth is also a result of decreased estrogen levels.

During menopause, which typically occurs between ages forty-five and fifty-five, your body starts producing even less estrogen. Estrogen replacement therapy is often recommended for preventing osteoporosis and for generally maintaining good health beyond menopause. In fact, studies show that women who take estrogen for up to ten years have a 37 percent lower risk of premature death.

HOW DO ESTROGENS WORK?

Some estrogens are produced by the hair follicles and may play a role in awakening follicles from their telogen phase and signaling them to enter their anagen, or growth, phase.

If you have a genetic predisposition to androgenetic alopecia, normal levels of estrogens will generally protect your hair from falling out. But if you are genetically predisposed and have low levels of estrogens, your hair may start to shed.

Estrogens are antiandrogens; they counterbalance and regulate androgens. In addition, estrogens are weak 5 alpha-reductase inhibitors. Thus, they interfere with the production of the enzymes required to convert testosterone into DHT and may guard against shedding.

HOW ARE ESTROGENS USED?

Topical and oral estrogens (usually formulations of estradiol) are often employed to help prevent hair loss in women but yield mixed results. They do not stimulate regrowth, but appear to stop the shedding caused by androgenetic alopecia.

During menopause, the dosage of estrogen required to preserve hair is higher than that currently prescribed to prevent osteoporosis. The two most widely prescribed estrogens are Premarin (Wyeth-Ayerst) and Estrace (Bristol-Myers Squibb). To halt hair loss, some physicians recommend a daily oral dose of Premarin (1.25 milligrams) or Estrace (2 milligrams).

In addition, some dermatologists have had success treating hair loss with a combination of topical estrogens and minoxidil. Discuss this option with your dermatologist.

ARE THERE SIDE EFFECTS?
According to the *Physicians' Desk Reference*, potential side effects of taking estrogen include vaginal bleeding, abdominal cramps, water retention, breast tenderness, headaches, depression, and nausea. More worrisome are an increased risk of gallbladder disease, greater chance of breast cancer, and blood clots in the legs and lungs.

NOTE: According to the *Physicians' Desk Reference*, before taking estrogen, check with your doctor if:
• You have ever had a bad reaction to estrogen.
• You have undiagnosed vaginal bleeding.
• You have breast cancer or any other estrogen-dependent cancer.
• You have any heart or circulation problems, including a tendency for abnormal blood clotting.

Finasteride (Propecia)

Originally developed to shrink an enlarged prostate and sold as Proscar, finasteride in lower doses has now been approved to treat baldness in men. This low-dose version is marketed as Propecia. Proscar and Propecia are manufactured by Merck. Studies in men indicate that it may grow back more hair than minoxidil does.

HOW DOES IT WORK?
Technically, finasteride is a 5 alpha-reductase inhibitor. It works by decreasing the production of one of the enzymes (5 alpha-reductase 2) required to convert testosterone into DHT, the hormone that triggers hair loss.

Merck has completed a clinical study of finasteride in postmenopausal women. In the study, forty-four women took finasteride, and fifty were given a placebo. After twelve months of treatment, the women using finasteride did not grow any hair.

The researchers and the manufacturer have concluded that finasteride is not effective in treating female androgenetic alopecia.

ARE THERE SIDE EFFECTS?
The *Physicians' Desk Reference* warns that finasteride should be used to treat male pattern baldness only. Because of the ability of 5 alpha-reductase inhibitors to interfere with the conversion of testosterone to DHT, finasteride may cause abnormalities of the external genitalia of a male fetus of a pregnant woman.

Thus, finasteride is not suggested for women of childbearing age due to its effect on hormone balances and possible birth defects. In fact, if you're pregnant or thinking about becoming pregnant, do not even touch a crushed finasteride tablet. Nor should you have intercourse with a man who is taking the drug unless he wears a condom. Finasteride can be transmitted to your body through semen.

Flutamide (Eulexin)
Flutamide is used in tandem with the drug Lupron to treat prostate cancer. Manufactured by Schering, flutamide has been studied in animals and humans as a potential antibaldness drug.

HOW DOES IT WORK?
A powerful nonsteroidal antiandrogen, flutamide blocks and weakens the action of androgens.

HOW IS IT USED?
The jury is still out regarding flutamide's effectiveness as an antibaldness drug. But in one study involving women, dosages of 250 milligrams taken twice daily in combination with an oral contraceptive produced modest hair regrowth.

ARE THERE SIDE EFFECTS?
According to the *Physicians' Desk Reference*, the drug has side effects that include anemia, anxiety, breast tissue swelling, diarrhea,

high blood pressure, and liver problems. In addition, your fetus may be harmed if you take flutamide while pregnant.

There is a newer nonsteroidal antiandrogen called bicalutamide (Casodex) used to treat prostate cancer. It is has fewer side effects than flutamide, according to medical research. Manufactured by Zeneca, bicalutamide has been mentioned on the Internet and elsewhere as a potential baldness remedy for women, although no research currently supports this use. As with flutamide, bicalutamide taken during pregnancy poses a potential hazard to the fetus.

NOTE: According to the *Physicians' Desk Reference*, before considering flutamide, check with your doctor if:
- You have liver disease.
- You are pregnant, plan to become pregnant, or are nursing.
- You are taking other prescription or nonprescription drugs.

Immunosuppressive Drugs

These drugs are used to prevent the immune system from rejecting transplanted organs. A side effect of treatment is increased hair growth, which is why these agents have been investigated as hair restorers, particularly in cases of alopecia areata.

HOW DO THESE DRUGS WORK?

By dampening the action of immune cells in the follicle, they may help halt the progression of alopecia areata.

The main immunosuppressive drug used to treat alopecia areata is cyclosporine, taken orally. It has been studied as a possible hair-restorer for numerous years. In Great Britain, scientists have tested oral and topical cyclosporine on a special kind of rat whose baldness is physiologically similar to that of alopecia areata—and with good results. The drug appears to convert damaged follicles to normal, hair-producing follicles.

Studies with people haven't been as promising. When cyclosporine was tested on humans in a 1987 study, the researchers used a topical preparation applied twice daily on fourteen patients suffering from extensive alopecia areata. The study lasted several months. By the end of the experiment, three patients had experienced normal hair regrowth.

Some researchers have tried combining cyclosporine with prednisone. In a 1997 study, eight patients (five women and three men) took 5 milligrams of cyclosporine per kilogram of body weight daily, along with 5 milligrams of prednisone. The dosages of cyclosporine were gradually reduced over a twenty-four-week period. By the end of the study, only two of the eight patients had cosmetically acceptable hair regrowth. The lowest dose of cyclosporine that produced these results was 3.5 milligrams per kilogram of body weight a day. Based on these results, the researchers noted: "Thus it does not appear that the use of low-dose prednisone increases the efficacy of cyclosporine. In addition, four of our eight patients had significant side effects."

If all else has failed, should you try cyclosporine as a last-ditch effort? Probably not. In 1992, the medical journal *Dermatology* related the case of a thirty-year-old woman who had tried everything, all to no avail. Suffering from alopecia since puberty, she was given oral cyclosporine daily for three months. Still, no hair regrowth.

ARE THERE SIDE EFFECTS?
The risk of using immunosuppressive drugs is high. With your immune system suppressed by these agents, you are at an elevated risk of infection and malignancies. High doses of cyclosporine may cause serious kidney damage, according to the *Physicians' Desk Reference*. If you've been previously treated with PUVA (see below) or anthralin, you are at an increased risk for skin malignancies.

Isoprinosine

Isoprinosine is a very old drug that has been tested extensively in other countries as an antiviral and antitumor agent. It appears to be beneficial in treating herpes, genital warts, influenza, HIV, and alopecia areata.

Isoprinosine is manufactured in Costa Rica but is not available in the United States. Many AIDS patients have traveled to Mexico to bring isoprinosine into the United States because it may be of some value in treating this dreaded immune disease. It's not a cure for AIDS, however.

HOW DOES IT WORK?

Research shows that isoprinosine is a powerful immune-boosting drug. To date, at least three scientific studies have looked into its effect on alopecia areata—all with positive results. In one of these studies, twenty-five patients were treated with isoprinosine for twenty weeks, followed by twenty weeks of treatment with a placebo. All of the participants had suffered from alopecia totalis for at least one year.

Eleven of the patients experienced new hair growth as a result of taking the drug. What's more, the drug enhanced their immunity. The researchers noted that isoprinosine "is a safe and effective therapy for certain patients with alopecia totalis."

ARE THERE SIDE EFFECTS?

Apparently, the drug has few, other than dizziness, slight stomachache, and itching.

According to the Life Extension Foundation, an advocate of alternative medicine, the FDA has said that it will not approve isoprinosine because its manufacturer promoted the drug's benefit for early-stage AIDS patients without first obtaining the FDA's permission.

Ketoconazole (Nizoral)

Ketoconazole is an antifungal drug available in tablets, as a cream, and as a shampoo. Manufactured by Janssen Pharmaceuticals, it is used to fight yeast infections, oral thrush, ringworm, and hard-to-treat fungal skin infections. Ketoconazole may also be helpful in treating androgenetic alopecia.

HOW DOES IT WORK?

Ketoconazole appears to interfere with the production of testosterone and acts as an anti-inflammatory agent—two reasons why it has been investigated for the treatment of androgenetic alopecia.

A 1998 study conducted at the University of Liège in Belgium found that ketoconazole shampoo used alone or in combination with minoxidil increased the size and density of hair, as well as shifted more hair follicles into their growth cycle. Investigators speculate that ketoconazole may reduce levels of testosterone around the hair follicles. Ketoconazole is a nonsteroidal agent.

Even though the findings of this study are good news, more research is needed to verify the results. Further, no tests have yet been conducted on ketoconazole tablets and their effect on baldness.

ARE THERE SIDE EFFECTS?

According to the *Physicians' Desk Reference*, side effects from using ketoconazole shampoo are extremely rare. A tiny percentage of people may experience itching, mild dryness of the skin, abnormal hair texture, and scalp irritation.

Potential side effects of taking ketoconazole tablets include abdominal pain, itching, nausea, and vomiting. Ketoconazole can interact dangerously with numerous other drugs. If you're taking other medications, be sure to let your physician and pharmacist know before combining ketoconazole with other drugs.

NOTE: According to the *Physicians' Desk Reference*, before considering ketoconazole check with your doctor if:
- You are allergic to the drug.
- You are pregnant, plan to become pregnant, or are nursing.
- You are taking other prescription or nonprescription drugs.

Liquid Nitrogen

Liquid nitrogen is a very cold liquid form of nitrogen gas that freezes on contact with the skin. Normally, it is applied to treat and remove warts, but it has been used as a treatment for alopecia areata.

HOW DOES IT WORK?

Liquid nitrogen is sprayed or daubed on the scalp until the skin freezes. The skin then thaws out, and after one or two treatments a week, there may be some hair growth.

ARE THERE SIDE EFFECTS?

The application of liquid nitrogen is not a widely used treatment for alopecia areata, and evidence is sketchy as to whether this type of therapy can successfully treat the disease. Some medical authorities believe it could do irreparable damage to skin cells.

Minoxidil (Rogaine)

If ever there was a "wonder drug" for baldness, minoxidil is it. Known popularly as Rogaine, minoxidil is one of two FDA-approved treatments for hair loss. It is the only antibaldness drug approved for women. If your hair loss is due to androgenetic alopecia—and it's just beginning—minoxidil is your best solution for stimulating regrowth.

Minoxidil was originally introduced as a medicine named Loniten to treat hypertension (high blood pressure). Quite by accident, its hair-growing benefits were discovered in the early 1970s when researchers noticed that hypertensive patients started sprouting extra hair. In 1980, the first such case was reported in the scientific literature. It described how minoxidil reversed hair loss in a man taking it for high blood pressure.

Some inventive researchers ground up minoxidil tablets, mixed the powder in a cream base, and applied the concoction to the bald spots of volunteers. In some, new hair took root. Interest in the drug intensified, and scientists began studying the drug as a potential baldness cure for both men and women. Today, minoxidil is the closest thing we have to a cure for baldness in women.

In the United States, minoxidil, marketed as Rogaine Regular Strength, was first approved as a prescription product for use by men in August 1988. The same product was approved for women in August 1991. It became available as an over-the-counter (OTC) medication in February 1996.

Two percent minoxidil is a generic over-the-counter drug, so you'll find it in numerous products now on the shelves of pharmacies, supermarkets, and health food stores. Some of these products include Equate 2%, Bausch & Lomb 2%, and Shen Min Activator.

A newer product, Rogaine Extra Strength for Men, was approved for OTC usage in November 1997, and approval of Rogaine Extra Strength for Women is expected soon. The extra-strength formulations contain a 5 percent concentration of minoxidil.

Five percent minoxidil products are available by prescription only. Costs vary, but the 2 percent solution can range from $8 to $10 a bottle. The prescription version is more expensive, costing from $30 to $45 a bottle.

HOW DOES IT WORK?

No one really knows for certain how minoxidil works to promote hair growth. Even so, there are some theories, based on scientific research. First, minoxidil is a vasodilator, meaning that it opens up blood vessels in the scalp. Blood can thus circulate more freely to the scalp and deliver more oxygen and nutrients to the hair follicles. The net effect may be to jolt hair follicles from their resting phase into their growth phase.

Second, minoxidil enlarges withered (miniaturized) hair follicles. Miniaturization occurs when androgens and other factors gradually shrink the hair follicles, choking off hair growth. By enlarging the hair follicle, minoxidil extends the life of the hair-growing cycle and gets hair growing again.

And third, minoxidil appears to promote cell division in keratinocytes, particularly those located in and around the hair follicle. Keratinocytes are cells that produce the hair protein keratin.

MINOXIDIL AND ANDROGENETIC ALOPECIA

Currently, minoxidil is the only medically approved treatment for women with androgenetic alopecia (hereditary hair loss). It appears to work very effectively for women. Here's a look at some of the research:

Regrows hair. The earliest studies on minoxidil were conducted in 1982 and 1983 by Upjohn, the makers of Rogaine. In clinical trials at twenty-seven medical centers across the country, a 2 percent solution of topical minoxidil or a placebo was given to 2,300 participants (mostly men and a few women), aged eighteen to forty-nine. The studies lasted four months, and by the end of the research period, 39 percent of the minoxidil group were showing new hair growth—some of it quite dense.

Studies with mostly women were conducted later. In 1993, Upjohn tested 2 percent minoxidil in a study of 294 women in ten centers throughout Europe. All suffering from androgenetic alopecia, the women were divided into a minoxidil group and a placebo group. The study lasted thirty-two weeks. Forty-four percent of those women in the 2 percent minoxidil group achieved new hair growth, compared to 29 percent in the placebo group.

A similar study was conducted in 1994 at the University of Texas in San Antonio. In eleven centers throughout the United States, 256 women (ages eighteen to forty-five) with androgenetic alopecia applied 2 percent minoxidil or a placebo to their scalps twice daily for thirty-two weeks. Approximately 63 percent of the minoxidil-treated women showed minimal to moderate regrowth. Those in the placebo group did not fare as well.

Increases scalp coverage. Topical minoxidil increases the number of hairs on your head, according to several well-designed studies.

At Duke University Medical Center in Durham, North Carolina, a 2 percent topical minoxidil solution applied twice daily significantly increased the number of normal hairs in women with androgenetic alopecia.

Similar results were found in a study conducted at the University of Texas Southwestern Medical Center in Dallas. In a trial of thirty-three women (aged twenty-two to forty-four) all with androgenetic alopecia, minoxidil produced minimal to moderate hair growth in about 60 percent of the patients.

To determine whether the drug could multiply the number of hair strands, researchers counted hairs on one-centimeter portions of the women's scalps. They found that, on average, the number of hair strands in these areas increased by nearly twenty extra hairs, thanks to minoxidil. (One centimeter is roughly the width of a small fingernail.)

Other studies have found that women using a 2 percent solution of minoxidil increased hair count by twenty-three to thirty-three hairs on areas of the scalp. Further, studies at Duke University have discovered that minoxidil can *double* the number of normal hairs seen on the scalp.

What these studies demonstrate is that the drug clearly multiplies the number of hairs on your head! None of the women using minoxidil in either of these studies experienced any side effects.

Thickens hair. Minoxidil beefs up your hair fibers, too. A 1988 study found that not only did topical minoxidil (3 percent solution) boost hair growth, it also widened the diameter of hair fibers in women. This made hair look thicker.

According to research conducted at the Kaiser Permanente Medical Center in San Francisco, a 2 percent topical solution of minoxidil increased hair weight by nearly 43 percent in women treated with the drug for thirty-two weeks, compared to only 1.9 percent for those treated with a placebo. The women who took part in the study were suffering from androgenetic alopecia.

Clearly, minoxidil is an effective weapon against androgenetic alopecia, but how well does it fight other forms of baldness? Numerous studies have looked into this, with mixed results.

Alopecia Areata

Minoxidil has been well tested in patients with alopecia areata, a disease characterized by total or patchy loss of hair. It is thought to be caused by an immune disorder.

In a study of forty-eight patients (which included twenty-six women), thirteen men and twelve women regrew hair while using a one percent topical solution of minoxidil. However, of these twelve women, only three experienced "cosmetically acceptable growth"—meaning that they no longer needed to wear a wig to conceal their hair loss.

Other studies have found that higher concentrations of minoxidil (3 or 5 percent solutions) appear to be more effective against alopecia areata.

Topical minoxidil, however, does not work well for severe cases of alopecia areata—those in which patients have lost most of their hair. A 1988 study at the Mayo Clinic showed that a 3 percent topical minoxidil solution applied twice daily to the scalp for a year produced very little hair regrowth in either men or women.

Medical experts generally agree that topical minoxidil is only somewhat effective in treating alopecia areata in both men and women. The less severe your hair loss, the better the treatment will work. Also, minoxidil often works better in combination with other agents, such as corticosteroids and anthralin, to treat alopecia areata (see below).

Chronic Telogen Effluvium

Minoxidil does not seem to be very effective against chronic telogen effluvium. In a few cases (observed in men only), topical minoxidil appeared to bring about telogen effluvium, and no one knows why. Once the minoxidil was discontinued, hair growth resumed and the shedding stopped.

Chemotherapy-Induced Hair Loss (Anagen Effluvium)
Minoxidil does not seem to reverse hair loss caused by chemotherapy, either. In a study of women beginning chemotherapy, a 2 percent solution of minoxidil applied twice a day did not prevent hair loss.

Other Types of Hair Loss
Nor does minoxidil work well for hair loss associated with nutritional deficiencies, thyroid disorders, diseases or conditions that scar the scalp, or the use of certain prescription medications.

MINOXIDIL AND OTHER ANTIBALDNESS REMEDIES
Minoxidil is being combined with other remedies to treat hair loss. These include tretinoin (Retin-A), finasteride (Propecia), azelaic acid, corticosteroids, and anthralin.

- Tretinoin (Retin-A) is a remedy for treating acne. Applied topically with minoxidil to the scalp, it appears to help regrow hair in many women. The active compounds in Retin-A are *retinoids*. They enhance the penetration and absorption of topical minoxidil into the hair follicles. For more information on Retin-A/minoxidil combinations, see below.
- Finasteride may also work well in tandem with minoxidil. Minoxidil sparks hair growth, while finasteride curbs hair loss. Although they work quite differently, together they potentially form a dynamic duo against baldness, which has led to the formulation of a lotion containing both. It is currently only available at selected pharmacies and some clinics.
  Finasteride is not recommended for women, however, because it can cause birth defects. You should talk to your dermatologist before using a minoxidil/finasteride combination.
- Azelaic acid has also been combined with minoxidil, in a product called Xandrox (see below). A dietary component of

whole grain cereals and animal products, azelaic acid has been shown to block the formation of DHT in the skin.

- Corticosteroids have been used with minoxidil to treat alopecia areata with fairly good results. In a sixteen-week study, topical 5 percent minoxidil with a topical corticosteroid (0.05 percent betamethasone) applied thirty to sixty minutes later produced fair to good regrowth in 56 percent of patients with alopecia areata. The minoxidil/corticosteroid combo worked better than either agent alone. Researchers speculate that the two drugs have a synergistic effect when used together, meaning that they strengthen and enhance each others' action.

  In addition, minoxidil appears to work well as a maintenance treatment to preserve hair growth after you have taken corticosteroids such as predisone. A study published in the *Archives of Dermatology* in 1992 found that 2 percent minoxidil helps prevent hair loss after you stop using corticosteroids.

- Anthralin may work well with minoxidil, too, particularly in the treatment of alopecia areata. In another study of alopecia areata patients, 5 percent minoxidil was applied twice a day, and anthralin was applied at bedtime, one or more hours after the second application of minoxidil. Patients applied the medications to their entire scalp. By week twelve, thirty-eight of the forty-nine patients using the combination had grown hair, and five patients had grown cosmetically acceptable hair by week twenty-four. With ongoing therapy, four of those five patients were able to maintain good hair growth for seven years.

HOW IS MINOXIDIL USED?

The drug is an easy-to-use, colorless, and virtually odorless liquid. Most minoxidil products come with both a dropper and spray adapter for controlled application. A dropperful contains just the right amount required for a single application. The pump sprayer requires just six pumps with each application. Some dermatologists discourage the use of the sprayer, however, because it delivers too much medication to the hair and not enough to the scalp.

Minoxidil should be used twice a day, once in the morning and once at night. Apply it directly to the thinning area of your scalp, then rub it in. Be sure your scalp is dry before use. Applying more than the recommended dose will not make minoxidil work any faster or better and may increase the risk of untoward side effects.

For best results, allow minoxidil to remain on your scalp for at least four hours before washing your hair, swimming, or going out in the rain.

If you miss an application, just continue on your regular dosage schedule. Don't try to make up for missed doses.

When using minoxidil, you don't have to change your normal hair-styling routine. However, apply minoxidil first and wait for it to dry before using hair spray, mousses, gels, and other hair care products.

The drug seeps down to the root of the hair follicle and awakens dormant, miniaturized follicles, reversing hair loss and stimulating these follicles to grow hair for a longer period of time. Initially, your new hair may be soft, downy, and colorless. But after continued use, minoxidil may promote the growth of new hairs the color and thickness of your original hair.

MINOXIDIL ENHANCERS

Minoxidil products are usually formulated in alcohol-based solutions. With long-term use, alcohol can dry out the skin, causing redness, itching, and flaking. Further, the skin on the scalp hardens, making it hard for minoxidil to fully penetrate and reach the hair follicles. Eventually, minoxidil doesn't seem to work as well as it did at first.

To solve these problems, a couple of companies are marketing "minoxidil enhancers" to help the medication better penetrate the skin. They work in numerous ways, either by restoring the skin of the scalp or by suspending the drug in a liquid state long enough for it to deeply penetrate the hair follicles.

The Minoxidil Enhancement System, developed by the DeYarman Medical Group, is a lotion containing polysorbate-80, which helps unclog pores. According to promotional materials from the company, the product decreases alcohol absorption to improve minoxidil's penetration into the scalp.

With this product, you mix your minoxidil with the enhancer and apply the required amount to your scalp. You should gently massage the solution into your scalp for about thirty to sixty seconds.

Another product is AMS9, distributed by Bio Trans. It contains citric acid, propylene glycol (a solvent that aids penetration), an antiseptic, and other ingredients. The product is designed to improve the health of the scalp so that minoxidil can better reach the hair follicles. Rather than mix it with minoxidil, you rub it on your scalp before applying minoxidil.

You should discuss minoxidil enhancers with your dermatologist to determine which product is most suitable for your particular situation, or whether you should even use one. Increasing the absorption of minoxidil may increase the chance of side effects.

WHEN WILL I SEE RESULTS?

With minoxidil, the first signs of hair growth are a thin "peach fuzz," but afterward, new hair is usually longer and thicker. Although some women see regrowth in just two to four months, it may take up to a full year of treatment to see whether minoxidil works for you. Shedding may stop in about two to four months. Minoxidil, however, does not work for everyone.

Hair regrowth typically lasts one year, and the amount of new growth is different for everyone. To maintain the benefits, continue to use minoxidil indefinitely. If you stop using it, your new hair and stabilized hair will fall out over the course of four to six months.

Now, suppose after one year of using minoxidil, it just doesn't work. There's no new hair, or the shedding has not stopped.

What next?

Discuss your options with your dermatologist. You may want

to pursue other treatments such as antiandrogens, which are often effective against long-standing, more severe, and more resistant cases of androgenetic alopecia.

ARE THERE SIDE EFFECTS?
The most common side effect is irritation of the scalp. In clinical trials, however, only 3 percent of regular users reported this problem. Some of the irritation may be caused by the propylene glycol in the solution, added to help the drug better penetrate the scalp. Other potential side effects include dry mouth and, in rare cases, lowered blood pressure and dizziness.

A rare side effect (occurring in 3 to 5 percent of women) is the growth of facial hair on the cheeks and above the eyebrow. This hair growth disappears with continued use.

Minoxidil appears to be quite safe when rubbed into the scalp. But because it is a vasodilator, meaning it expands the blood vessels, it should not be used by anyone with heart disease.

Minoxidil has not been linked to sexual problems or birth defects. It should not be used, however, if you are pregnant or nursing. The long-term safety of the drug is not known.

NOTE: According to the *Physicians' Desk Reference*, do not use minoxidil if:
- You are sensitive to or have had an allergic reaction to the medication.
- You use other topical prescription medications on your scalp. (Check with your physician.)
- You are pregnant or nursing.
- You are under eighteen.

Proxiphen
Available by prescription only, Proxiphen is a formulation containing the drugs minoxidil, phenytoin, tretinoin (Retin-A), and spironolactone (Aldactone). Promotional information on the

product states that it "grows significantly more hair on more people than any other agent."

Proxiphen was developed by Dr. Peter H. Proctor, who is not only a medical doctor but also a pharmacologist. He also developed a nonprescription version of the formula, Proxiphen-N, which is described on pages 105–106.

HOW DOES IT WORK?

Each of the pharmaceuticals in Proxiphen promotes hair regrowth by its own individual mechanism. Minoxidil, for example, appears to awaken hair follicles from their resting phase, enlarge withered (miniaturized) hair follicles, and promote cell division that leads to hair growth. Phenytoin is an anticonvulsive medication known to produce hair growth as one of its side effects. Tretinoin activates cell division, and spironolactone is an antiandrogen that interferes with the production of DHT. Together, these drugs may work more effectively than either agent used alone.

HOW IS IT USED?

The medications in Proxiphen are suspended in a cream base. After washing and drying your hair, apply a dab of the cream on areas of hair loss. Apply the product only once a day, morning or evening.

To obtain the product, you must be under the care of a physician who has appropriately diagnosed your hair loss. You'll need to produce one of the following: a copy of a minoxidil prescription written to you for the treatment of hair loss, a copy of your medical records or a copy of a doctor's office receipt listing hair loss as a diagnosis, or a note from your physician stating that you have hair loss. In addition, you must consult with Dr. Proctor by phone regarding your particular case, or have your physician write a prescription for Proxiphen.

For information on Proxiphen and other products, visit Dr. Proctor's website at www.drproctor.com.

According to information posted on the above website, side effects are rare. About 2 percent of the time, some patients may experience an allergic skin reaction to the formulation.

PUVA (Psoralens and Ultraviolet Light)

PUVA, also known as phototherapy, is used to treat alopecia areata. With this treatment, you ingest a "psoralen," a light-sensitive drug, and then undergo a short exposure to ultraviolet light. Sometimes topical psoralens are applied. Treatments are given over a three- to six-week period, usually two to three times a week for six months, or until hair regrowth occurs. Each treatment takes three to five minutes. You wear eye-protection with ultraviolet-blocking glasses while undergoing treatment.

HOW DOES IT WORK?

PUVA is believed to work by suppressing the immune system. PUVA treatment of alopecia areata has been researched for more than twenty years. Scientific studies show that PUVA:

- Appears to work well against alopecia areata, regardless of how long you have had the disease.
- Is usually not effective against alopecia universalis.
- Has an overall success rate of 40 to 60 percent.
- May provide long-standing relief from alopecia areata. Some patients relapse after treatment but many do not.

ARE THERE SIDE EFFECTS?

PUVA has few side effects, although the treatment may cause nausea. However, PUVA may promote skin cancer in susceptible individuals, making this treatment less than an ideal choice.

Spironolactone (Aldactone)

Spironolactone is a drug used to treat high blood pressure. It is classed as a diuretic because it increases the elimination of sodium and water from the body. Spironolactone, however, does not cause potassium loss. For this reason, the drug is technically termed a "potassium-sparing diuretic." Spironolactone is manufactured by Searle and sold as Aldactone. Some dermatologists prescribe it to treat androgenetic alopecia.

HOW DOES IT WORK?

Spironolactone counteracts the action of aldosterone, a hormone that regulates the body's salt and potassium levels. It is also a powerful antiandrogen that works in two ways. First, it slows down the production of androgens in the adrenal glands and ovaries. Second, it blocks the action of androgens. Like three riders trying to hop on the same cab, spironolactone, testosterone, and DHT all compete for entry into the cells of the hair follicle. Spironolactone muscles the two androgens out of the way.

Ultimately, both actions interfere with the conversion of testosterone into DHT, the culprit in hereditary hair loss and thinning. Consequently, spironolactone halts hair loss and produces meaningful hair regrowth in some people.

So far, only a few studies have been conducted on spironolactone as a hair-loss remedy. One of these involved seven women who took 200 milligrams of the drug every day for a year. Six of the women regrew their hair. Despite the lack of medical studies, many dermatologists prescribe it for women with androgenetic alopecia, often in combination with an oral contraceptive.

HOW IS IT USED?

As a treatment for hair loss, spironolactone is taken orally or applied topically. Oral doses usually range from 100 to 200 milligrams daily for a year or two. Afterward, the dose may be gradually reduced. Many patients report improvement within six months of use.

In certain cases, spironolactone may be a part of a treatment regimen that includes estrogen therapy and 2 percent topical minoxidil. Consult your dermatologist as to whether you should use spironolactone in this manner.

In addition, spironolactone is an ingredient in a topical formulation called Proxiphen (see pages 71–73) designed to treat baldness in men and women. This product also contains minoxidil, Retin-A (tretinoin), and other ingredients. Anecdotal evidence indicates that it appears to stop hair loss, thicken hair, and regrow lost hair. It is available by prescription. You can obtain more information on the product by visiting the following website: www.drproctor.com.

ARE THERE SIDE EFFECTS?

Because it blocks the action of testosterone, spironolactone may produce certain side effects in men, including decreased sex drive, impotence, and breast enlargement. For these reasons, balding men are usually prescribed the topical version only. Women, however, can take the oral version, with fewer problems.

According to the *Physicians' Desk Reference*, spironolactone may cause menstrual problems such as menstrual irregularity and midcycle bleeding. Other side effects include breast tenderness, abdominal cramps, digestive problems, and fatigue. If you take spironolactone, report any untoward reactions to your physician.

NOTE: According to the *Physicians' Desk Reference*, do not use spironolactone if:
- You have kidney or liver disease.
- You are pregnant, plan to become pregnant, or are nursing. (Spironolactone may expose the fetus to unnecessary harm. In addition, the drug appears in breast milk.)
- You have trouble urinating.
- You have high blood potassium levels.
- You are taking other medications, such as potassium supplements or ACE (angiotensin-converting enzyme) inhibitors.

Thymopentin

Thymopentin is a synthetic version of the hormone thymosin, secreted by the thymus gland. Tested widely in Europe, thymopentin is used to treat rheumatoid arthritis, skin disorders, various infectious diseases, and alopecia areata. Thymopentin is taken only by injection, because intestinal enzymes destroy the drug before it can be absorbed.

HOW DOES IT WORK?

Thymopentin may work well against stubborn alopecia areata. A group of researchers in Italy selected thirty-seven patients who had not responded to treatment for alopecia areata and divided them into two groups. These patients received either intradermal injections (into the affected scalp sites) or intravenous injections of thymopentin for four weeks. The patients had alopecia areata over more than 50 percent of their scalp and had suffered from the disease for at least two years.

Of those receiving intradermal injections, two had complete hair regrowth within six months, four had partial regrowth, and eight (two with patchy alopecia and six with alopecia totalis or universalis) did not respond.

In the intravenous group, three had complete regrowth of their hair within six months, and eight (five with patchy alopecia and three with alopecia totalis or universalis) had partial regrowth. When the treatment was repeated six months later in those who did not have complete regrowth, one grew new hair and three had partial regrowth.

THYMOPENTIN AND OTHER ANTIBALDNESS REMEDIES

The same researchers also experimented with a combination treatment—thymopentin and squaric acid dibutyl ester (SADBE), discussed on the next page. Twelve patients received intravenous injections of thymopentin and topical treatment on the left side of the scalp with SADBE. Five patients (one with alopecia totalis and four with alopecia areata affecting more than 50 percent of the scalp) experienced complete regrowth by six months. Six others had partial regrowth, and one patient, who had alopecia universalis, did not respond at all.

Based on their findings, the researchers noted that thymopentin, injected intravenously or intradermally or used with SADBE, can be beneficial for treating severe alopecia areata. Further, they believe that thymopentin may improve the results of SADBE.

ARE THERE SIDE EFFECTS?
According to an article published in the medical journal *Transgenica*, the drug produces few adverse side effects, with the exception of sleep disturbances and fatigue, and is well tolerated by patients.

Topical Contact Sensitization Therapy
"Topical contact sensitizers" describe a trio of chemicals that block the faulty autoimmune reaction thought to be responsible for hair loss in alopecia areata. The three contact sensitizers used most often are: dinitrochlorobenzene (DNCB), squaric acid dibutyl ester (SADBE), and diphenylcyclopropene (DPCP). All can be effective against alopecia areata, particularly when the disease affects 50 percent or more of the scalp. Patients with 100 percent hair loss (alopecia totalis and alopecia universalis) do not respond as well.

HOW DO THEY WORK?
These chemicals are actually irritants, or allergens, that, when applied to the scalp, activate an allergic reaction that causes renegade immune system cells to retract from the hair follicles, possibly reactivating hair growth.

HOW ARE THEY USED?
A solution containing the contact sensitizer is applied to your scalp by a dermatologist. You'll be instructed to not wash your hair for several hours or even a few days. Your dermatologist will

probably advise you to cover your scalp when outdoors and protect it from the sun for six to forty-eight hours, since sunlight degrades the medicine.

Initially, applications are usually administered once a week. Your dermatologist may reduce the frequency of the applications, depending on the sensitivity of your skin and your response to treatment.

WHEN WILL I SEE RESULTS?

When treatment is successful, cosmetically acceptable hair growth appears within about twenty-four weeks. If you don't respond by then, your doctor will probably discontinue contact therapy.

Topical contact sensitizers have been studied extensively for at least thirty years. Here is a brief overview of what researchers have discovered about these agents, including potential side effects:

DNCB. With weekly applications, DNCB can stimulate new hair growth within three weeks to six months. In one study, patients with long-standing alopecia totalis regrew new hair within eight weeks after receiving weekly applications of DNCB. Further, women seem to respond better to DNCB therapy than men do. And in some cases, DNCB is more effective than injections of triamcinolone acetonide.

DPCP. In Great Britain, DPCP is the treatment of choice for alopecia areata. Generally, treatment produces cosmetically acceptable results in approximately 40 to 60 percent of the patients who try it. DPCP does not work as well if you have chronic alopecia totalis, however. Some of DPCP's side effects include eczema, blisters, and sleep disturbances, according to medical research.

SADBE. If you've had alopecia areata for a long time, SADBE may be an appropriate therapy to try. Research shows that it may work against long-standing alopecia areata. On average, it may take between five and twenty weeks of treatment to see new hair growth. SADBE is well tolerated, with few side effects, according to medical research.

Tretinoin (Retin-A)

Quite probably, you know "retinoids" best as the nutritional supplements vitamin A and beta-carotene, or the acne medication Retin-A, also known generically as tretinoin or retinoic acid.

Some retinoids are naturally derived from vitamin A, a nutrient that is essential for growth, vision, and the health of the skin. Vitamin A has been used as a therapeutic agent in dermatology for more than fifty years.

Other retinoids are chemical copies, or synthetic versions, of the natural forms. Both the natural and synthetic agents have the power to successfully treat numerous conditions, from acne to psoriasis. They work inside the nucleus of the cell, aiding in growth and cellular reproduction.

Tretinoin, marketed as Retin-A and Renova by Ortho Dermatological, was one of the first synthetic retinoids to be developed. It is available as a topical ointment used to treat acne. More recently, tretinoin has been in the dermatological spotlight for its ability to erase facial wrinkles and rejuvenate the skin.

Another big plus for tretinoin: According to medical studies, it helps stimulate hair regrowth.

HOW DOES IT WORK?

Tretinoin activates cell division. Medical research into the action of tretinoin has discovered that it helps promote hair growth at the cellular level. It increases the cellular concentrations of a special protein that is allowed access to cells. Once inside the cell nucleus, this protein hooks up with tretinoin. The bond they form promotes protein synthesis and cell division, leading to hair growth.

Tretinoin prolongs the hair-growing cycle. Research exploring the role of retinoids and hair growth began in the 1980s. In animal studies, vitamin A–deficient hairless gerbils treated with topical tretinoin started growing new hair. Other animal studies found that tretinoin alone and in combination with minoxidil could prolong the anagen, or growth, phase of the hair follicle, and decrease its resting period (the telogen phase).

Studies with animals are one thing, but what about humans? So far, the research looks just as promising. In 1986, a study of fifty-six people with androgenetic alopecia showed that topical tretinoin (a 0.025 percent concentration) promoted meaningful hair regrowth in 58 percent of the patients. One of the women in the study had suffered from severe alopecia for more than twenty years. Amazingly, she started growing new hair after using tretinoin for only eighteen months!

Tretinoin enhances the action of minoxidil. The same study also looked into the effect of a tretinoin-minoxidil (5 percent solution) combination on hair growth. After one year, the combination therapy produced normal hair regrowth in 66 percent of the patients who used it. Scientists believe that tretinoin enhances the absorption and penetration of minoxidil into the hair follicles.

More recently, a landmark study was conducted on the benefits of this combo, and the results are truly amazing. For two years, 2,210 patients suffering from either androgenetic alopecia and alopecia areata were tracked while using a proprietary formula—a precise blend of 2 percent minoxidil and 0.025 percent tretinoin applied as a hair spray. The formula was developed by a New York City physician Dr. Adam Lewenberg, who has pioneered the combination of minoxidil and tretinoin for treating baldness.

Remarkably, 90 percent of the patients who sprayed the formula on, four times a day, showed visible—even cosmetically acceptable—hair regrowth after just three months of use. Of the patients who continued to use the formula for one and a half to two years, 91 percent had grown beautiful, normal hair, according to the study. Some of these patients had tried other medical treatments, without success, but were able to regrow normal hair by using this formula. The only people who did not respond were men who had been losing their hair for more than twenty years.

The strongest results were seen in women. According to the newsletter *National Women's Review*: "Currently, no other treatment, whether it is medical or non-medical, can come close to the success established in this study for treating women's hair thinning and hair loss problems."

Tretinoin promotes the health of the sebaceous glands. Other medical studies have found that tretinoin helps regulate the function of sebaceous glands. Tretinoin sees to it that the sebaceous glands surrounding the hair follicle do not overproduce sebum, which is an oil that lubricates your hair. Sebum contains DHT, the hormone that shrivels hair follicles, bringing on hair loss. Over time, too much DHT in the scalp can destroy hair follicles. By moderating the secretions of the sebaceous glands, tretinoin helps control DHT levels in the skin and prevents hair loss.

TRETINOIN/MINOXIDIL PRODUCTS

Currently, formulations of tretinoin with minoxidil are available by prescription only. There are several places you and your dermatologist can contact to obtain the product, if not available at your local pharmacy:

- Adam Lewenberg, M.D., 184 East 70th Street, New York, NY 10021; 212–249-8800 or toll-free 1–888-HAIR-133. Dr. Lewenberg is the well-known hair-loss expert who formulated a topical treatment consisting of 0.025 percent tretinoin and 2 percent minoxidil in a convenient 2-ounce spray bottle.

  According to his promotional literature, Dr. Lewenberg encourages patients to see him at least once in his New York office. However, if that's not possible, you can telephone him for a free consultation to start the treatment. He asks that you photograph the front and top of your head before treatment begins and once every three months afterward so that he can evaluate your progress. Also, you should call Dr. Lewenberg every three months and follow the medication instructions exactly as given.

The cost of the treatment is $60 to $70 per bottle (depending on how many bottles you purchase at a time), plus $10 for shipping and insurance. You must order a minimum supply of six bottles. Dr. Lewenberg offers a vitamin/mineral supplement as well, which is recommended as a complementary treatment. The supplement costs $10 a bottle.

For more information, visit Dr. Lewenberg's website at www.baldspot.com.

- Community Drug (www.communitydrug.com or www. minoxidil.com). This product comes in a solution of either 2 percent or 5 percent minoxidil, plus 0.025 percent tretinoin. It costs $32 to $35 a bottle, depending on the quantity you order, and requires a prescription.

- Central Iowa Compounding, 4132 University Avenue, Des Moines, IA 50311; 515–274-4464. This product is formulated with 5 percent minoxidil and 0.025 percent tretinoin. Available in a spray pump, the product costs $45 a bottle and requires a prescription.

- Re-Mox: This formulation is available by prescription only from Physicians Hair Growth. The women's formula contains 3 percent minoxidil and 0.025 percent tretinoin. Before ordering this product, you must first have a telephone consultation with one of the Physicians Hair Growth doctors. The number is 1–800-99 HAIR 44. For more information on the product and how to order it, visit the group's website at: www.physicianshairgrowth.com.

HOW IS TRETINOIN USED?

The available research on tretinoin for the treatment of baldness indicates that it works best on androgenetic alopecia. Little is known about whether it can help with other forms of baldness.

Tretinoin should be used at night—for two reasons. First, sunlight can degrade tretinoin. And second, tretinoin may make your skin overly sensitive to sun, and your scalp could get severely sunburned.

ARE THERE SIDE EFFECTS?

With initial use of tretinoin, you may experience temporary hair loss, according to medical reports. Although rare, this condition occurs because tretinoin breaks apart the chemical bonding between skin cells. Hair in the telogen (resting) phase thus comes out more easily. But in about three months, new hair will grow in, and the good news is that this hair will be thicker.

In some people, scalp irritation may occur with use. However, this may subside with continued treatment as your scalp becomes used to the medication. If not, you may want to discontinue treatment.

If you work in an occupation with considerable sun exposure, be sure to cover tretinoin-treated skin areas well.

NOTE: According to the *Physicians' Desk Reference*, do not use tretinoin if:

- You have any type of skin disease affecting your scalp.
- Your scalp is red, inflamed, infected, or otherwise irritated.
- You are sensitive to or have ever had an allergic reaction to tretinoin.
- You are pregnant or plan to become pregnant.
- You are lactating. (It is not known whether the drug appears in breast milk.)

Xandrox

Xandrox is a formulation containing a 5 percent concentration of minoxidil, a 5 percent concentration of azelaic acid, and beta-methasone valerate, an anti-inflammatory drug.

HOW DOES IT WORK?

The potential antibaldness actions of Xandrox are attributed to minoxidil, which fights hair loss in numerous ways, and azelaic acid, shown in scientific research to stifle the formation of follicle-damaging DHT in the skin. The two drugs may exert a synergistic benefit in fighting baldness.

HOW IS IT USED?

Xandrox is applied topically to a dry scalp, either by medicine dropper or by spray. The medication should be used twice a day for four months or longer. There is a nighttime version of Xandrox formulated with 0.025 percent Retin-A. Xandrox was developed by Richard Lee, M.D., of Regrowth, Inc., and is available by prescription only.

Regrowth, Inc. expects to launch a prescription formula containing a 12.5 percent concentration of minoxidil, 5 percent azelaic acid, and 0.025 percent betamethasone valerate. For more information on these products, visit the following website: www.minoxidil.com.

ARE THERE SIDE EFFECTS?

The package insert that comes with Xandrox notes that the formula may produce some skin irritation due to the various pharmaceutical agents found in the product.

Zinc (Prescription Doses)

Given in prescription, therapeutic doses, the mineral zinc may help regulate the immune system to help alter the course of alopecia areata. High doses are required, however, and may cause vomiting and diarrhea. Talk to your doctor about whether you should take extra zinc as supplemental therapy for alopecia areata. For more information on zinc, see page 152.

Hair Savers: What the Experts Recommend

Jean-Claude Bystryn, M.D.
Professor of Dermatology, New York University School of Medicine
Medical Advisory Board of the National Alopecia Areata Foundation (NAAF)

Dr. Bystryn is engaged in research on understanding the causes of hair loss in alopecia areata and is particularly interested in the possibility that it results from an immune reaction against hair follicles.

For women just beginning to experience alopecia areata, Dr. Bystryn advises the following:

"The best first-line treatment of early alopecia areata restricted to a few lesions is injections of cortisone into sites of hair loss. The cortisone medication used most often is called Kenalog. It is injected directly into sites of hair loss. Because each injection covers only a small area, multiple injections usually need to be given to sufficiently cover an area of hair loss. There is only slight discomfort associated with the treatment. Normally, the treatment is repeated every three to four weeks. If no hair growth is observed after three or four injections, then you need to discuss alternate treatment options with your dermatologist."

Hair Savers: What the Experts Recommend

Wilma F. Bergfeld, M.D., F.A.C.P.
1992 President of the American Academy of Dermatology
Head of Dermatology, Clinical Research and Dermatopathology at the Cleveland Clinic

Dr. Bergfeld is a leading authority on hair loss and specializes in its treatment. Here are her recommendations on treating alopecia areata:

"The scope of alopecia areata is broad, ranging from minor to severe. Commonly associated with other autoimmune diseases, alopecia areata should be identified by personal and family history, as well as by laboratory screening tests. These tests should include antinuclear antibody (ANA) and thyroid screening test to include T4, TSH, and the Microsomal antibody test (to exclude Hashimoto's Thyroiditis).* Alopecia areata is strongly associated with allergies and a skin condition known as vitiligo. Characterized by chalky white patches of skin framed by a dark border, vitiligo is a disorder of pigment-producing cells in the skin. It may be related to a thyroid problem or on autoimmune disorder."

(continued on page 86)

(continued from page 85)

According to Dr. Bergfeld, basic therapy for alopecia areata should include:

- Psychological support of patient and family
- The use of camouflage techniques, including scarves and wigs. (Prescriptions can be written to allow for deduction as a medical expense. However, it is rare that insurance companies will cover this expense.)
- Antiseborrheic shampoo one to three times a week
- Ultraviolet light (sun) therapy
- Topical anti-inflammatory drugs such as topical steroids
- Nutritional supplements such as a multiple vitamin/mineral formula

Dr. Bergfeld also advises combination therapy using:

- Oral antihistamines for allergy symptoms
- Topical tars or anthralin (1 percent), applied for thirty minutes or left on all night, one to seven days a week
- Topical prescription cortisone preparations, one to seven times a week
- Sensitization therapy as an immune modulator
- PUVA (Psoralen and UVA light)
- Cortisone injections

"Like androgenetic alopecia, alopecia areata is best diagnosed and treated by a dermatologist, a physician who specializes in hair, nail, and skin disease."

*A disease in which the body becomes allergic to its own thyroid hormone. Hashimoto's Thyroiditis is a common cause of underactive thyroid and goiter (a swelling of the thyroid gland).

PART 3

Fallout
Shelter

FIVE

Fighting Baldness: Commercial Nondrug Treatments

W ITHOUT A DOUBT, drugs can work wonders in the treatment of hair loss, and when used appropriately, they have enormous value. But these medicines may not be your first choice. Depending on your particular condition, you may want to try a nondrug treatment first (but only with your dermatologist's blessing), or as a complement to drug therapy. Nondrug preparations are used to treat various types of hair loss, from androgenetic alopecia to alopecia areata.

A handful of studies have found that certain nondrug lotions, creams, sprays, or other external products promote hair regrowth and can reduce shedding. But by law, manufacturers of these products cannot market them as true hair-loss remedies. If they did, they'd have to file a new drug application with the FDA and prove that the product is effective—a requirement that involves controlled clinical trials and millions of dollars in research expenses.

Keep in mind that the only two products officially approved by the FDA for hair loss are the drugs minoxidil and finasteride (Propecia).

Although a lot of nondrug preparations have not been widely tested, they may be worth a try. But weigh the evidence carefully before buying. To help decide, here's an alphabetical list of some of the leading nondrug commercial treatments on the market.

Aminexil (Dercap)

This antibaldness treatment is manufactured by L'Oreal/Vichy Labs and is available only in Europe.

WHAT'S IN IT?

Aminexil contains a patented "anti-fibrosis molecule" that is structurally related to minoxidil and reported to stimulate hair growth, according to company literature. There are two versions of the treatment, one formulated for men and the other for women. The women's product contains vitamins B_6 and B_5 (pantothenic acid).

HOW DOES IT WORK?

The manufacturers of Aminexil believe that hair loss is linked to the accelerated aging of the hair root, characterized by *fibrosis*, or the overproduction of collagen. Fibrosis makes the roots overly rigid, and this compresses the blood vessels that feed and stimulate them. As a result, the roots weaken and hair falls out prematurely. Aminexil appears to fight the process of fibrosis by interfering with the action of an enzyme involved in making collagen. By combating fibrosis, Aminexil helps preserve the health of the hair roots and prevent hair loss.

In a clinical trial involving 160 women, more than 60 percent showed a decrease in hair loss, and more than 80 percent grew stronger, thicker hair. In addition, clinical tests in three European hospitals demonstrated that the product preserves 10 percent more hair than a placebo. Aminexil certainly looks promising, and there are no reported side effects from its use.

HOW IS IT USED?

The suggested use is three vials a week for two months. Follow the manufacturer's instructions for application.

WHAT DOES IT COST?

Aminexil costs about $42 for a six-week supply. There is an Aminexil shampoo as well, and it costs approximately $11.

WHERE CAN I BUY IT?

Although the treatment is only available in Europe, you can order it from Pharmaworld International Mail Order Pharmacy at www.pharmaworld.com.

Anagen3

Manufactured in Italy but available by mail order in the United States, Anagen3 is a nondrug topical lotion that has enjoyed tremendous popularity in Europe. The product is made by Anagen Laboratories of Italy.

WHAT'S IN IT?

Anagen3 contains "acid polysaccharides." These are starchy, gelatinous carbohydrates that people with thinning hair often lack.

HOW DOES IT WORK?

Anagen3 does not claim to regrow hair, but the product may retard hair loss and fortify existing hair by replenishing it with polysaccharides, according to company literature. Studies at the University of Milan have found that it is effective in penetrating dormant hair follicles and restoring essential nutrients. People who use Anagen3 feel that it strengthens and thickens the hair shaft. In a poll of Anagen3 users, 86 percent said there were satisfied with the results.

HOW IS IT USED?

You use Anagen3 in two phases. In the first phase, you apply the product daily for twenty-four days; in the second phase, you apply it every other day for forty-eight days. Some people have experienced good results after just two weeks of the treatment.

WHAT DOES IT COST?

One kit (twenty-four vials) costs approximately $89.95. You'll need to purchase two kits to use the product as recommended. The product comes with a money-back guarantee.

There are Anagen3 companion products, including a medicated shampoo, a moisturizing shampoo, conditioner, and hair spray. These range in price from $8 to $15.

WHERE CAN I BUY IT?

In the United States and Canada, you can order Anagen3 by mail through Lifestyle Fascination, 1935 Swarthmore Avenue, #3023, Lakewood, NJ 08701; 1–800-669–0987.

Crinagen

Developed by Raztec Enterprises of New York City, Crinagen is a doctor-formulated, all-natural scalp preparation applied topically. It can be used by both men and women. Crinagen does not claim to promote hair regrowth. However, the natural ingredients in the product may provide some benefit if you have thinning hair.

WHAT'S IN IT?

Crinagen is a blend of natural ingredients—including zinc, saw palmetto, B-complex vitamins, and ginkgo biloba—polysorbate 20, and glycerine. Polysorbate 20 is thought to clear hair follicles clogged by DHT, secretions, and other irritants. In addition, glycerine and polysorbate 20 help dissolve the other ingredients and ferry them into the hair follicles.

HOW DOES IT WORK?

The product is positioned as a natural alternative to finasteride and minoxidil. Two of its ingredients—zinc and saw palmetto— are believed to attack DHT in much the same way finasteride does: by blocking the activity of the enzyme 5 alpha-reductase, which converts androgens into DHT. Research into saw palmetto and prostate disease shows that the herb does indeed block this enzymatic reaction. Thus, it can be argued that the herb may do the same in androgenetic alopecia. Further, zinc has been shown to hamper the action of 5 alpha-reductase in human skin. (For more information on oral supplementation with saw palmetto, see page 168; for information on oral supplementation with zinc, see page 152.)

Crinagen also contains two B-complex vitamins, vitamin B_6 and niacin. Vitamin B_6 works together with zinc in blocking 5 alpha-reductase, and niacin triggers the release of histamine. Histamine is a naturally occurring compound in the body that dilates blood vessels, so that more blood and nutrients can be delivered to the hair follicle. Medical experts speculate that increasing the blood supply to the hair follicle may increase its size and possibly reverse the miniaturization caused by DHT. Ginkgo biloba, another herb in Crinagen, also increases blood supply to cells, including those of the hair follicle. (For more information on oral supplementation with ginkgo biloba, see page 163.)

HOW IS IT USED?

Crinagen should be sprayed on all balding and thinning areas one to three times a day. Each application consists of four to five sprays.

You can use Crinagen with other baldness treatments, including minoxidil and Retin-A. In addition, you can use the product with hair spray, mousse, and gel, but let it dry for at least ten minutes before applying other hair preparations. Certain shampoos are recommended for use with Crinagen, and these include Nizoral (ketoconazole, available by prescription only) and T-Gel, manufactured by Neutrogena.

According to company literature, you may see some results within one to four months. These results may include hair regrowth in some people. More often, Crinagen retards hair loss. Some people may get no results at all.

WHAT DOES IT COST?
Each 4-ounce bottle costs approximately $19.95 and should last from one to three months, depending on the number of daily applications used.

WHERE CAN I BUY IT?
You can order Crinagen from the manufacturer's website: www. raztec.com.

Fabao 101D
Dubbed a "magic liquid for hair," this botanical blend (also called Dabao) was developed by Dr. Zhao Zhangguang, a Chinese doctor trained in herbal medicine. According to articles in *Newsweek* and the *New York Times*, Dr. Zhao began his quest for a baldness cure in 1973 after a woman schoolteacher who was bald came to him for help. Even though she wore a wig, she was ostracized and made fun of in her community because of her baldness. Sympathetic, Dr. Zhao began working in earnest, whipping up 101 various herbal blends before he found the right formula. He tried it on a patient who was bald but was being treated for a fever and skin rash. The concoction did not heal the fever, but it did cure the baldness!

In 1976, a Chinese reporter (who also happened to be bald) investigated the remedy, tried it, and started regrowing hair within three months. He wrote an article about it, and word spread throughout Asia. By 1986, Dr. Zhao had set up a factory in Beijing to mass-produce the remedy, called 101 Hair Regeneration Liniment.

Today, Dr. Zhao runs more than fifty factories in China, all churning out hair and skin care products. At least seven hospitals in China have used the original formula to treat androgenetic alopecia and alopecia areata. Dr. Zhao's original hair-restoring product is marketed worldwide as Fabao 101D. In Chinese, *fabao* means "precious hair."

WHAT'S IN IT?

The herbs in Fabao 101D include ginseng, safflower, mulberry leaves, stemona root, fruits of the pepper plant, sesame leaves, Chinese angelica, ginger, walnut meat, a type of acontitum (or monkshood), and a type of salvia (sage). The product has an alcohol and water base and is recommended for men and women in the early stages of androgenetic alopecia.

Some of these plants, particularly angelica, contain plant chemicals that in tiny amounts have a healing effect on the skin. In folk medicine, sage has a reputation as a hair-restorer, one with the ability to halt hair loss and preserve hair color. In Asia, sage extracts are common ingredients in hair rinses and shampoos. In Chinese medicine, safflower is thought to be a "vasodilator," meaning that it opens blood vessels and thus helps more nutrients reach the hair follicles. Ginseng is believed to stimulate blood circulation and thus is good for the scalp.

HOW DOES IT WORK?

In Asia, many medical doctors feel that hair loss is caused by poor blood supply to the scalp, malnourished hair roots, sebum-clogged pores, and the presence of DHT in the hair follicles. According to promotional literature from Fabao 101D, the product counters each of these problems. It restores healthy blood circulation to the scalp, dilates the blood vessels that feed hair follicles, regulates sebum secretions in the scalp, and corrects the problems caused by DHT. The net effect is to revitalize dormant hair follicles, grow healthy hair, and preserve existing hair.

Several years after developing the product, Dr. Zhao tried it on more than a thousand patients in Beijing with a success rate of 90 percent. Since then, the product has been scientifically tested with results published in European, Japanese, and Chinese medical journals.

In 1987, the product compared favorably to another hair-restorer in a test involving 109 people. Eighty-three percent of those using Fabao 101D reported good results.

Conducted in 1994, a test on rats, guinea pigs, and rabbits, whose hair had been shaved, showed that Fabao 101D significantly increased the weight of regrown hairs in the shaved area. This finding indicates that the product may thicken hair.

To date, the only other significant study was conducted with men suffering from androgenetic alopecia. In this well-designed study, 396 men were divided into either a treatment or placebo group. They massaged it onto a warm, dry scalp twice a day for four to five minutes. No one knew whether they were using Fabao or the placebo.

The researchers took hair counts every two months to see whether any new hair had sprouted. In addition, a six-member panel made up of professionals familiar with baldness judged the cosmetic results. Finally, the participants were asked their opinions on how well the remedy worked.

Based on these three measurements, the study noted that the treatment produced a modest effect on the growth of normal hair. The researchers concluded that Fabao can increase hair growth by an average of twenty-four to twenty-nine hairs per 5-centimeter area over a period of six months.

However, those using the placebo also regrew a significant amount of hair! How could that be?

There are numerous explanations, say the researchers. First, the density of your hair depends on the season of the year. Hair is not as dense in November, but grows gradually thicker as spring and summer approach. This study started in September and ended in April. Second, many of the participants may have enrolled in the study during a time when much of their existing hair was in its growth phase. Third, warming and massaging the scalp (as required) to apply the preparation could have had a stimulating effect on hair growth. Fourth, it is possible that much of the hair growth as observed by the panel and participants was vellus hair.

Certainly, this is a significant study—one that shows the promise of nondrug treatments. Hopefully, more research will be conducted, particularly involving women.

HOW IS IT USED?
The product comes as a thin lotion that you apply to the thinning areas of your scalp once a day. It is suitable for both men and women. In rare cases, the product may cause potential side effects, including an irritated scalp and inflamed follicles, according to one published research study.

The manufacturer says that, on average, users should see results in eight weeks, although it may take as long as six months.

WHAT DOES IT COST?
Fabao 101D comes in 3.4-ounce bottles, and each bottle lasts six to eight weeks. For most people, the cost is between $30 and $46 a month. By purchasing the product in bulk, you pay less.

There are other formulas too: 101G for patients in the late stage of hair loss; 101F for patients with oily scalps in the late stage of hair loss; and 101 Shampoo.

WHERE CAN I BUY IT?
You can purchase Fabao 101 formulas by accessing the website—www.fabao.com—or by calling toll-free 1–800–229–8587. The formulas come with a thirty-day guarantee. If not satisfied, you may return the products within thirty days for a full refund. (Shipping and handling costs are not refundable.)

Folligen
This doctor-invented product is a nondrug treatment designed to improve scalp health, a necessary prerequisite for healthy hair growth. Folligen was developed by Loren Pickart, Ph.D., an expert in human aging, wound and bone healing, and hair growth.

He has received more than one hundred patents on various classes of pharmaceutical agents for tissue regeneration. Because many men with high androgen levels never go bald, Dr. Pickart believes that hair loss is not directly related to androgens but rather to poor skin health.

The company that markets and manufactures this product is Skin Biology. One of its advisers is Professor Hideo Uno, a leading researcher on hair growth. Dr. Uno conducted much of the early research on minoxidil.

WHAT'S IN IT?

According to company literature, this product contains a patented copper-peptide complex called Ancilin, along with various herbs and nutrients. This copper complex forms a protective barrier over the skin and helps manufacture superoxide dismutase (SOD), an antioxidant enzyme that inactivates certain free radicals believed to damage hair follicles. Free radicals are unstable molecules that bore through cell walls and make it easy for disease-causing agents to slip in and do often-irreparable harm.

HOW DOES IT WORK?

Available as a lotion or cream, Folligen works on the principle that poor skin health is the ultimate cause of hair loss, and clinical studies of the product show that it does improve skin.

Folligen's copper peptides, which are bonds of copper and amino acids, are believed to help increase the number of blood vessels supplying the follicles. More nutrients can thus reach the follicles, resulting in thicker, healthier hair growth. Also, copper-peptides appear to plump up fat cells surrounding the hair follicle. Some investigators feel that these fat cells support the health of the follicle. Increasing their size may enhance follicle health.

Promotional material from Skin Biology states that the product works best in women forty to seventy years of age, may stop hair shedding within a month or two, may thicken the hair shaft, and may restore hair growth in some people.

Folligen helps repair any minor skin damage or irritation from using tretinoin (Retin-A) or other topical antibaldness medications. It may also be effective for restoring scalp health following hair transplantation and for repairing scalp damage caused by dyes, permanents, and other chemical treatments, according to the manufacturer.

HOW IS IT USED?

The manufacturer recommends its 2-Step Hair Growth System, in which you use a 2 percent minoxidil solution, along with Folligen (applied at bedtime and washed out the next morning). The rationale is that minoxidil promotes hair growth, while Folligen improves scalp health. Folligen is also recommended for use with a combination of minoxidil and tretinoin (Retin-A) therapy.

Folligen has a loyal legion of users who feel that it reduces hair loss, prevents scalp flaking, and soothes scalp irritations caused by other baldness treatments. As one woman put it, "My husband says my hair is looking much thicker and better."

WHAT DOES IT COST?

Folligen costs approximately $17.95 for a 2-ounce tube of either the cream or lotion. It lasts from thirty to forty-five days when applied about four times a week.

WHERE CAN I BUY IT?

You can purchase Folligen by calling 1–800–405–1912 or accessing the website: www.skinbio.com.

Foltene

Developed by Crinos, an Italian pharmaceutical company, Foltene is a line of products marketed to improve scalp and hair health. The line includes a topical scalp treatment, as well as a hydrating shampoo, a deep-cleanse shampoo, a conditioner, a gel treatment, and a nutritional supplement.

WHAT'S IN IT?

The Foltene Professional Topical Scalp Treatment and other products in the line contain a patented ingredient called Tricosaccaride, a formulation of six protein-carbohydrate compounds found naturally in hair. The scalp treatment, shampoo, conditioner, and gel also contain vitamins, amino acids, and herbs.

HOW DOES IT WORK?

Some researchers believe that certain types of hair loss are caused by abnormal blood circulation in the scalp skin, as well as sebum-clogged pores that choke off the oxygen supply to the hair follicle, leading to its destruction. The protein-carbohydrate compounds, they speculate, unclog pores and promote better blood circulation to the scalp. Further, some early experiments with these compounds showed that they may increase the sulfur content of the hair follicles and stimulate the production of keratin.

In addition, in a study published in 1963, a group of Italian researchers treated thirty bald patients with Foltene and found that the product increased hair growth, halted shedding, and reduced excessive sebum and dandruff.

In 1987, a study was published in the *Journal of Korean Medical Science* that gave a thumbs-up to Foltene, too. The researchers conducted three different trials to test the product's effectiveness. First, they applied Foltene on seven men and three women suffering from androgenetic alopecia. Treatment continued for twenty weeks, and half of the patients regrew their hair. Hair shedding was reduced by 70 percent, on average. The study does not indicate who fared better—the men or women.

In the second trial, the researchers tested the effects of Foltene on thirteen patients (two men and eleven women) with alopecia areata. More than half the patients had hair regrowth.

Seven patients (two men and five women) participated in the third test. They were suffering from what the researchers called "seborrheic alopecia," in which the sebaceous glands overproduce sebum, causing baldness. Again, the results were in Foltene's favor. Most of the patients regrew their hair, and the product reduced sebum production considerably.

There were very few side effects from using the product, although a few patients experienced some itching and scalp irritation.

Based on their findings, the researchers concluded that "Foltene shows a remarkable therapeutic value for male pattern baldness, alopecia areata, and seborrheic alopecia."

HOW IS IT USED?

When using Foltene products, you are instructed to shampoo with the deep-cleanse shampoo first, then towel dry your hair. Apply one vial of the topical scalp treatment and gently massage it into your scalp. Leave the treatment on and style your hair using the gel. The hydrating shampoo can be used alternatively with the deep-cleanse shampoo. The conditioner can be applied after shampooing but is not recommended for use on days when the topical treatment is applied.

WHAT DOES IT COST?

The topical treatment costs approximately $12.85, and the shampoos cost $7.95 each. The conditioner and gel are $5.99 each.

WHERE CAN I BUY IT?

You can purchase Foltene products from various websites. One of these is www.sn2000.com.

Kevis

Quite probably you have heard Kevis advertised on the radio. Imported from Italy, Kevis is a patented lotion promoted to improve hair health. There is also a Kevis shampoo designed to be used with the lotion. Kevis was developed in Italy and is now available in the United States.

Kevis contains hyaluronic acid, a natural gel-like substance distributed in human sperm and other body tissues of humans and animals. Hyaluronic acid, which helps maintain moisture levels in hair, is found in a number of hair care products.

Kevis is also formulated with B-vitamins (biotin and pantothenic acid); thioglycoran, a type of carbohydrate; and thurfyl nicotinate, a vasodilator.

HOW DOES IT WORK?

Some hair-loss experts theorize that hyaluronic acid penetrates the hair follicle and forms a protective shield around it, sealing off the DHT receptors. That way, DHT can't latch onto cells and destroy the hair follicles.

Numerous studies have been conducted on Kevis, mostly in Europe. This scientific research has found that Kevis:

- Decreases percentage of hairs in the resting (telogen) phase.
- Decreases hair shedding.
- Nearly eradicates the presence of DHT in the hair follicle.
- Increases hair in the active growth phase.
- Builds hair body and fullness.
- Improves scalp health.

If you have lost some hair following childbirth, Kevis may be of some value. In a study of fifty women (between twenty and thirty-five years of age) who lost hair after having babies, Kevis helped restore hair growth and prevented further hair loss—and did so in about thirty-six days.

Also, Kevis may slow down hair loss caused by chemotherapy, according to one study. Sixty-one patients undergoing chemotherapy were divided into two groups; half the group used Kevis, while the other half (the control group) did not. Those in the Kevis group experienced a much slower rate of hair loss than the controls did. Further, the use of Kevis helped restore scalp health following chemotherapy.

HOW IS IT USED?

Apply the lotion in the morning or at bedtime to wet or towel-dried hair and massage into the scalp. Leave the lotion on for a minimum of four hours or until the next time you shampoo your hair. After applying the lotion, you may feel a warm, flushed sensation on your scalp. This is normal and occurs because Kevis stimulates circulation in the tiny blood vessels feeding the hair follicles. The sensation should subside in about thirty minutes.

After two weeks or so of using the product, you may see some improvements in the quality of your hair and the health of your scalp. It takes about three months of use for full improvement, correction of scalp disorders such as dandruff and seborrhea, and reduced hair breakage.

WHAT DOES IT COST?

To obtain information on prices, call 1–800–242–0999 and ask to speak to a Kevis consultant.

WHERE CAN I BUY IT?

You can order Kevis products by calling 1–800–242–0999.

Nisim New Hair Biofactors

On the market since 1993, Nisim New Hair Biofactors is a group of products designed to control hair loss and restore your hair's normal growth cycle. The products are manufactured by Nisim International of Brampton, Ontario, Canada, and include an herbal extract, shampoo, spray conditioner, finishing conditioner, and an oil-free conditioner.

WHAT'S IN IT?

The herbal extract's main ingredient is the herb saw palmetto. The extract also contains the amino acids cystine, cysteine, and methionine, all important hair proteins; B-vitamins (pantothenic acid, inositol, and biotin); and natural vasodilators to stimulate scalp circulation. (The shampoo contains many of the same ingredients.)

The extract is available in two formulas: one for oily hair and scalp; the other for dry hair. The extract for dry hair contains hyaluronic acid, which helps hair retain moisture.

HOW DOES IT WORK?

To date, the extract and shampoo have been tested only in men—with a success rate of 85 percent in those who used it consistently for five to six months. The men regrew normal hair, and in some cases doubled or tripled hair regrowth. Another study in men found that the extract and shampoo reduced DHT in the follicles.

Nisim International says that the deep-cleansing scalp shampoo removes oil, sweat, dirt, and excess sebum—plus controls excessive hair loss within days. The company also notes that the shampoo may help control hair loss following childbirth.

The manufacturer sent me a sample of the shampoo, and I tried it. My hair felt and looked thicker and was very easy to manage. It is an excellent product that does not leave your hair feeling filmy and weighted down like many regular shampoos do.

HOW IS IT USED?

You should use the herbal extract two to three times a day—after washing your hair with NISIM shampoo. The company says in its promotional literature that you should see results in three to six months.

WHAT DOES IT COST?

A two-month supply of these products costs approximately $49.95.

WHERE CAN I BUY IT?

If you are interested in trying these products, the company has a toll-free number—1–800-65NISIM—or you can purchase the products at certain hair salons. NISIM products can also be ordered from www.madison-avenue.com/nisim1.htm.

Proxiphen-N

This product is a nondrug topical formulation developed by Peter H. Proctor, Ph.D., M.D., who holds seven patents for the treatment of hair loss. Dr. Proctor also developed Proxiphen, a prescription medication that contains minoxidil, phenytoin (an anticonvulsive medication known to produce hair growth as one of its side effects), tretinoin (Retin-A), and spironolactone. For information on Proxiphen, see pages 71–73.

WHAT'S IN IT?

Proxiphen-N contains agents believed to help stimulate hair growth. One of the key agents is superoxide dismutase (SOD), an antioxidant enzyme that neutralizes free radicals. Manufactured with the help of copper, zinc, and manganese, SOD has been found to reduce stress-induced hair loss in animals and prevent hair loss as a result of radiation therapy. Proxiphen-N also contains a copper peptide (a copper/protein combination), which may enhance hair growth, and nitric oxide, a messengerlike substance that may signal hair to start and keep growing.

HOW DOES IT WORK?

The ingredients in Proxiphen-N may have a possible synergistic effect that boosts hair health. The product is certainly worth a try, especially since Dr. Proctor is a recognized authority on hair health. Proxiphen-N can also be used with minoxidil. You may also want to try Proxiphen-N's companion products, NANO shampoo and NANO conditioner.

HOW IS IT USED?

Follow the manufacturer's recommendations for dosage and application.

WHAT DOES IT COST?

Proxiphen-N costs $59.95 for a two-month supply and $109.95 for a four-month supply. For a two- to three-month supply, NANO shampoo costs $39.95; a two-month supply of the conditioner is $29.95. These products all carry a time-limited, money-back guarantee.

WHERE CAN I BUY IT?

To order Proxiphen-N and other products, visit Dr. Proctor's website: www.drproctor.com.

Rhodanide Replenisher

Rhodanide Replenisher is a line of hair care products that includes a hair revitalizer as well as a shampoo and hair rinse. The revitalizer is a solution applied topically to improve the appearance, thickness, and condition of your hair. It has been tested in Europe as a potential hair-restorer.

WHAT'S IN IT?

The active ingredient in these products is rhodanide, or thiocyanate, a natural saltlike, sulfur-containing substance that is a constituent of hair. Rhodanide also plays a role in metabolism, enzyme reactions, and cell division.

HOW DOES IT WORK?

According to information from the product's distributor (NHF Distribution, Inc.), rhodanide strengthens the keratin structures of the hair strand. Absorbed into the hair, the substance helps protect hair from chemicals, detergents, pollutants, the sun, and other environmental factors. It also helps hair retain more moisture. The net effect is shinier, healthier hair, with more body and bounce.

Interest in rhodanide as a hair-restorer was sparked after studies with sheep and mink showed higher wool production and stronger fur quality when the animals were given rhodanide. It has also been studied in guinea pigs, whose hair supposedly resembles human hair. In that study, it increased the hair's growing cycle.

In 1997, German researchers published their findings on rhodanide as a potential remedy for androgenetic alopecia. For six months, physicians treated 102 men with a retail product (Activogland) containing rhodanide, or with a placebo. Use of the product prolonged the growing cycle of hairs and reduced the number of hair follicles in the resting stage. About 80 percent of the participants in the treatment regrew hair, and about half of those had sustained their hair growth a year later.

Most of the physicians who participated in the study gave the product good ratings. It is unclear from the scientific literature and product information whether there will be further studies of rhodanide's effect on hair loss in men or women.

HOW IS IT USED?

The distributor of Rhodanide Replenisher advises using the revitalizer two or three times a week. Wash and lightly towel dry your hair first, then apply the solution so that it coats all your hair. Massage it into your scalp but do not rinse it out. Dry and style your hair.

Both men and women can use this product. You should experience healthier, easier-to-manage hair with initial and continued use, according to the distributor. Although the products are not marketed as hair-growth stimulants, the distributor also states that normal hair growth may begin after a month of treatment and becomes more apparent after three months of use.

WHAT DOES IT COST?

The shampoo costs about $39; the revitalizer, $69; and the rinse, $42.

WHERE CAN I BUY IT?

These products are sold through NHF Distribution, Inc., to beauty salons or for home use under various brand names: Rhodanide

Replenisher, Rhodanide Activance, Activogland, and Preluderm. You can purchase them online by accessing the distributor's website: www.rhodanide.com. The distributor also has a toll-free number: 1–800-880–8065.

Semodex/Nioxin

Launched in April 1998, Semodex is a line of products manufactured by Nioxin, a therapeutic hair care company. Semodex products include a shampoo (Semodex Sebolytic Cleanser), a rinse (Semodex Stabilizing Rinse), and a topical ointment (Semodex Serum). They were created in response to research that found a link between thinning hair and a common microscopic mite known as *Demodex folliculorum*. This mite is present in the scalp and hair follicles. It lives off the oily secretions of the scalp and produces a harmful enzyme called lipase that may contribute to hair thinning. The mite by itself does not cause hair loss.

Demodex is believed to appear during adolescence and is present in almost all adults by middle age. Apparently, the use of regular shampoos, conditioners, and antidandruff products does not remove the lipase produced by the mite.

WHAT'S IN IT?
Nioxin formulates its products with a number of natural ingredients. These include natural sugars called "mucopolysaccharides," biotin, niacin, ginseng, saw palmetto, and superoxide dismutase (an antioxidant enzyme).

HOW DOES IT WORK?
In a study conducted by Nioxin researchers, lipase was discovered in the hair follicles of fifty men and women with thinning hair. Lipase damages the condition of the hair and scalp. Removing its buildup helps create fuller, thicker, and healthier hair, according to Nioxin.

The Semodex serum is designed to prevent lipase from accumulating on the scalp, while the shampoo washes away the lipase that already exists on the scalp and in the hair follicles.

Nioxin makes other products for men and women with thinning hair. These include cleansers, hair conditioners and moisturizers, a styling gel, hair sprays, a booster, and two dietary supplements. Some women feel that using Nioxin products helps restore hair lost after childbirth.

HOW IS IT USED?
Semodex hair care products are designed to be used daily in conjunction with each other. Follow the manufacturer's suggestions for application.

WHAT DOES IT COST?
Semodex products range in cost from $9.95 to $39.95. Other Nioxin products cost between $7.95 and $49.99.

WHERE CAN I BUY IT?
Nioxin's hair care products are available exclusively through salons worldwide. You can also order them by calling their toll-free number—1–800-915–0230—or through the company's website: www.nioxin.com.

Thymu-Skin

Thymu-Skin is a topical solution that is massaged into the scalp. According to product information, Thymu-Skin may halt baldness and regrow hair by boosting the immune system. A faulty immune system is believed to be the cause of at least one form of baldness, alopecia areata.

WHAT'S IN IT?
This product is formulated with a granular extract containing thymosin, the principal hormone of the thymus gland. The

thymosin found in Thymu-Skin is obtained from the thymus glands of calves. The product also contains aloe vera, vitamins, and the herbs nettle and birch.

HOW DOES IT WORK?

The action of Thymu-Skin is based on the fact that the thymus gland shrinks as we age. Located in the chest just behind the breastbone, this gland secretes thymosin, a hormone vital to the health of the immune system.

Many scientists believe that our slowly disappearing thymus gland is related to the aging of the immune system. One of the side effects of deteriorating immunity may be baldness. Theoretically, by resupplying our bodies with thymosine, we can prevent age-related baldness—and even strengthen our immunity.

The thymus-calf extract in Thymu-Skin is a natural form of thymosin. There is also a synthetic derivative of the hormone known as thymopentin. It has been tested extensively for many years in Europe as a therapeutic agent for treating patients with rheumatoid arthritis, skin disorders, various infectious diseases, and alopecia areata. It shows good results in all these areas of disease. For more information on thymopentin, see pages 76–77.

You can't take thymopentin or natural thymus-calf extract orally because intestinal enzymes destroy them before they can be absorbed. Thymopentin is thus given by injection; Thymu-Skin, by massaging into the scalp.

Thymu-Skin's formulation is approved as a cosmetic by the FDA and by similar authorities in Canada and Germany.

HOW IS IT USED?

The hair revitalizer should be applied to the scalp twice a day for four weeks, then once a day for six to eighteen months. Thereafter, use it twice a week. The shampoo should be used twice a week.

WHAT DOES IT COST?

There are two Thymu-Skin products on the market: Thymu-Skin Hair Revitalizer at $69 a bottle, and Thymu-Skin Biologically Active Hair Shampoo at $39 a bottle. Each bottle provides a six-week supply.

WHERE CAN I BUY IT?

Thymu-Skin is distributed by Superclean Distributors, Inc., phone: 954-484–1291; fax: 954-733–2091.

Tricomin

Tricomin is a line of hair care products developed by ProCyte Corporation for men and women with thinning hair. The product line includes a spray (Tricomin Solution Follicle Therapy Spray), shampoos (Tricomin Revitalizing Shampoo and Tricomin Conditioning Shampoo), and a conditioner (Tricomin Restructuring Conditioner).

WHAT'S IN IT?

The chief ingredient in these products is a copper peptide, a patented blend of copper and essential amino acids (proteins). Copper is vital to hair health. In fact, healthy hair follicles are rich in this mineral.

HOW DOES IT WORK?

During the hair's growth cycle, the follicle needs copper to help support growth. One way to deliver an ample supply of copper to follicles is through the scalp by applying a topical solution like Tricomin. When bound to proteins as a copper peptide, copper is better absorbed into the follicles and surrounding areas, according to product information. Research has shown that copper-peptide solutions do increase hair counts.

HOW IS IT USED?

Wash and condition your hair with one of the Tricomin shampoos and conditioners. Let your hair dry. Then apply the spray. The products should be used daily.

WHAT DOES IT COST?

Costs vary, depending on where you purchase the products.

WHERE CAN I BUY IT?

Tricomin products can be purchased at hair salons or by calling their toll-free number: 1–800-548-HAIR.

NOTE: Prices of products described in this chapter may change. Consult the manufacturer or distributor for a current price list.

SIX

Passport to Thicker-Looking Hair: Cosmetic Treatments

W HILE TREATING hair loss, how should you care for your hair on a day-to-day basis? Tender loving hair care is vital to minimize the shedding and enhance overall hair health. Fortunately, the development of hair care products for fine hair, and for those with hair loss, is advancing at a rapid pace. Many of these products are designed to make your hair look thicker, fuller, and healthier. What follows is a rundown of products and styling techniques to consider.

Shampoos

Shampooing not only keeps your hair clean, it can also complement treatments for hair loss. Generally, the product you choose should be a mild one, with a minimum of chemicals. Also, look for shampoos containing silicone derivatives such as "dimethicone" and "dimethicone copolyol." Products with these ingredients do a good job of building hair volume in people with thinning hair.

If your hair is shedding, it's best to use a therapeutic shampoo designed for treating hair loss. Progaine Shampoo, for example, is formulated to be used with Rogaine (minoxidil). Many of the nondrug lotions, extracts, and revitalizers described in the previous chapter are marketed as part of a line of products that includes therapeutic shampoos.

With these special shampoos, carefully follow directions for use. But always check with your dermatologist to see which therapeutic shampoos you should use.

You may have to switch shampoos from time to time, however. There's a bona fide condition known as "shampoo fatigue" in which a shampoo builds up on your hair, deposits a residue, and fails to leave hair clean and shiny. A product known as a "clarifying shampoo" will rid your hair of this buildup. Use it two or three times, then resume using your regular shampoo.

Here are some guidelines for proper care when shampooing and drying your hair:

- Gently shampoo your hair.
- Shampoo oily hair every day, or else it will look even thinner. Here's why: Daily washing removes not only dirt and residue from hair products but also excess sebum. Sebum tends to make your scalp shine, and a shiny scalp makes bald areas look more exposed. (Wash less often if your hair is naturally dry.)
- Lightly massage your scalp for about thirty seconds while shampooing. This will help promote scalp circulation and improve the overall health of your hair.
- Rinse your hair well. Shampoo can leave a residue that draws dirt and irritates the scalp.
- If using a blow dryer, towel dry your hair first. Then set the dryer on warm or cool.
- Be gentle to your hair when it's wet. Wet hair can stretch about a third of its length and thus can be easily broken or damaged. Untangle it first with your fingers and let it dry a bit before combing or brushing.

Conditioners

Consider using a conditioner. Damaged hair is negatively charged. Conditioners contain ingredients that are positively charged.

Thus, they bind to hair, making it stronger, softer, and more resilient. Plus, they coat the hair shaft so that it feels thicker or fuller, but only temporarily. Conditioners can also protect your hair against damage due to brushing, blow drying, and hot rolling.

The key is choosing a conditioner that is right for your type of hair. Dry hair needs a moisturizing product, for example. Fine, limp hair requires a lightweight conditioner. Generally, the fewer ingredients listed on the label, the lighter the conditioner. Ask your hair stylist to recommend products that complement your hair type, or consider a therapeutic conditioner formulated specifically for hair loss and hair thinning.

Conditioners come in various forms. Rinse-out conditioners are applied after you shampoo, left on for about sixty seconds, then rinsed off. If your hair is fine, avoid moisturizing conditioners because they tend to flatten hair. A lightweight rinse-out conditioner is preferable; it can help detangle your hair, making it easier to comb.

Leave-in conditioners are applied to wet hair and are not washed off. They detangle hair and give it shine. Some leave-in conditioners are specially formulated to enhance body. Generally, foam leave-ins work best for fine hair.

Deep conditioners are left on hair for up to thirty minutes, then shampooed off. They restore shine, resiliency, and softness to damaged hair.

Hot-oil treatments soften dry hair but are not recommended for fine hair because they can make it limp.

Root Lifters

Containing strong resins and plant extracts, these products are applied to the base of your hair to prop up it up at the roots. They lift but without creating stiffness, and this effect gives the illusion of fuller hair.

You should apply the root lifter on wet hair before you begin styling. Most products have special spouts, making the lifter easy to apply.

Examples of root lifters include: J.F. Lazartique Root Volum-nizer, Graham Webb Styling Root Infusions, and Catwalk Root Boost.

Volumizers

When more than a thousand women were polled in a department store, 72 percent perceived their hair as fine, thin, and lacking in body. Volumizers to the rescue! These products also contain resins but work differently than root lifters do. Volumizers coat each individual hair fiber, swell the cuticle, and double its width. Your hair looks thicker and fuller as a result.

Spray the volumizer over your wet hair before styling. Some products come as gels or creams that are applied to wet hair before blow-drying. Examples of volumizing products include Rusk Thick and Paul Mitchell Volumizing Spray.

Shampoos and conditioners also contain volumizing ingredients. These include keratin, collagen, and cosmetic carbohydrates. They coat the hair shaft, strengthening hair and giving it more bulk.

Cosmetic carbohydrates are made from wheats and plant sugars and are used as ingredients in conditioners. They have been found in laboratory tests to strengthen hair, particularly after blow-drying. They also coat the hair shaft, making it shinier and easier to comb.

Swell Perms

Ask your hairdresser about a "swell perm," a mild permanent wave designed to give the illusion that hair is thicker than it really is.

If you are considering a perm, ask for one that uses acidic waving lotions. These have the gentlest action and are recommended for fragile hair.

Perms work best when hair is in good condition to begin with. The same is true of hair coloring. Consult your dermatologist before deciding whether to have a perm.

Hair Coloring

If you have dark hair, try a lighter color. Lightening your hair reduces the contrast between your hair color and scalp color, disguising balding areas and making them less noticeable. Color, in general, adds body and weight to hair. In addition, highlights give the appearance of greater volume.

When coloring your hair, avoid products formulated with peroxide and ammonia. Both can damage your hair and scalp, causing hair to break off and become thin. Peroxide, in particular, assaults keratin, along with hair color, and the result is weakened hair. Consult your dermatologist before deciding whether to color or highlight your hair.

Products to Avoid

Some gels and mousses tend to weigh hair down and clump individual strands together. Balding areas thus become more noticeable, and hair looks thinner. Stick to styling products that make your hair look fuller. Finding the right products may require some experimentation.

Brushing and Styling

To protect your hair and minimize further shedding, follow these guidelines for brushing and styling:

- Use a wide-tooth comb rather than a brush. In fact, too much brushing can damage your hair's outer layer, so forget your mother's advice about giving your hair one hundred brush strokes a day.
- If you do use a brush, select one with natural bristles; they effectively soak up hair's natural oils and redistribute them over the rest of the hair. Natural-bristle brushes also do a better job of removing dust and dirt from hair. In addition, brushing and combing help increase circulation to the scalp.
- Minimize excessive tension when using any type of hair curler. Wind curlers loosely.

Hair Cuts

Fine, thin hair looks best with a short blunt cut, perhaps with some layering around the face. This style makes your hair look thicker, less patchy, and is easier to care for.

A skilled stylist will know how to cut and style your hair according to your pattern of thinning. Do some research to find a hair care professional with experience in cutting thinning hair.

In addition, keep your hair trimmed as needed, particularly the ends. Split ends can advance right up the hair shaft, creating more damage.

Quick Fix for Balding: Cover-Up Products

Want fuller-looking hair with fewer bald patches peeking out? Then try camouflaging—the art of concealing thin areas with cover-up products. These are cosmetic products that provide a temporary, quick-fix solution to bald spots and thinning hair. Fortunately, these products have come a long way since the messy spray-ons introduced years ago.

TOPPIK AND COUVRé

Among the new generation of cover-ups is Toppik, a complex of tiny, microfiber hairs made from the same keratin found in real hair. Manufactured by Spencer Forrest Products, Toppik is neither a spray nor cream. Simply shake the canister gently, and in seconds, thousands of hair fibers begin merging with your own hair. Charged with static electricity, they bond with your hair and stay securely in place—even when you're sleeping or out in wind or rain, according to the manufacturer. The product does not smear or stain, either.

For both men and women, Toppik is designed to look natural and undetectable. Available in six shades, it is compatible with minoxidil and works well with hair transplants. You wash it out with shampoo.

One regular-size canister costs $19.95 (a 30-day supply); the economy size costs $39.95 (a 75-day supply). There's an optional hair spray, Toppik Fiberhold Spray, which is formulated to increase the bond between the fibers and your hair. It costs $9.95 for a 120-day supply; and $4.95 for a 30-day supply.

Spencer Forrest Products also makes COUVRé Protein Hair Expander. The company says that movie and television stars have used the product for the past fifteen years to enhance hair. According to company literature, it's recommended by dermatologists because it makes transplanted hair look fuller. Several major textbooks have endorsed COUVRé for this application.

COUVRé is not really a cover-up, but a special protein-based formula that penetrates the hair fiber to help make it thicker. The company says the product expands each fiber by up to 50 percent and that you'll see an increase in the thickness of your hair the very first time you use it.

COUVRé can be used with minoxidil and other topical solutions as long as you apply the expander afterward. The product is not greasy or gummy, and will not rub off or stain, according to the manufacturer.

There's also a COUVRé Thickening Shampoo designed to remove the buildup of sebum and other elements that can make hair look limp. There is also a COUVRé Alopecia Masking Lotion that covers up scalp show-through. It is applied with a little sponge.

Available in eight shades, COUVRé costs $36.95. You can use it with Toppik and other Spencer Forrest products.

You can order these products or obtain more information by calling 1–800–416–3325.

DERMMATCH

DermMatch is a powdered formula that has been used by dermatologists and hair transplant surgeons for years. Here's how it works: Using a special applicator, rub it directly on thinning areas of your scalp. The product then begins to coat and thicken each individual hair nearby. You can still brush your hair, even swim with it on, according to DermMatch, Inc., the manufacturer.

In addition, DermMatch has received endorsements from journals and magazines that report on hair-loss issues.

The product comes in a convenient little disk similar to packaged eye shadow. Each disk costs $29.95 and will last about one year. DermMatch is available in seven shades. You can even blend two colors to get the right match for your hair color. According to the manufacturer, the product is nongreasy, nor will it clog your pores.

You can order the product by calling 1–800-826–2864 (United States and Canada), or 1–301-208–9060 (International).

MAKE YOUR OWN COVER UP

Before spending money on a cover-up product, try making your own. You can color in or lightly shade bald spots with powdered eye shadow or an eye shadow crayon that matches the color of your natural hair. This technique makes the thinning less noticeable.

SEVEN

Electrical Stimulation of Hair Growth

YOU'RE PROBABLY familiar with electrolysis—the cosmetic process in which electrical impulses kill unwanted facial hair down to the root and keep it from growing back. But did you also know that there is another electrically based technique designed to do the opposite—get hair growing again?

Called ElectroTrichoGenesis (ETG), this technique is based on electrical stimulation of the scalp. It is different from electrolysis, though. With electrolysis, a current is directly applied to the skin, whereas ETG utilizes a noncontact electrostatic field that surrounds the scalp.

Electricity has been used for a long time in medicine to enhance bone healing and soft tissue repair. Interestingly, a side effect of some of these treatments has been hair regrowth. A company named Current Technology Corporation, headquartered in British Columbia, Canada, applied this knowledge to the development of a treatment for androgenetic alopecia.

In 1996, the company launched this technology after ten years of testing. It now holds the worldwide patent on ETG and has received government approval from health regulatory agencies in Canada, New Zealand, Australia, and Mexico. The treatment, however, is not available in the United States. Already, more than fifty thousand treatments have been administered to balding patients throughout the world.

ETG Treatments

Treatments are given in clinics. With each treatment, you recline in a special chair that's fitted with a beauty salon hair dryer-type hood. The hood is placed over your head so that its inner disposable lining, which contains electrodes, is about 5 centimeters from your scalp. This hood delivers low-intensity, evenly distributed electrostatic pulses to your scalp. Nothing touches your scalp or body; the treatment is painless and noninvasive. It is recommended that you receive weekly treatments. Each twelve-minute session costs $25 to $50.

What the Research Shows

ETG is not a cure for baldness, but it does seem to effectively treat androgenetic alopecia, as verified by scientific research. In fact, three major scientific studies have looked into the effectiveness of ETG.

Back in 1990, researchers at the University of British Columbia School of Medicine in Vancouver, Canada, administered the treatment to thirty balding men over a period of thirty-six weeks. There was also a control group of twenty-six men who received treatment from what appeared to be an identical device but in fact emitted no electrical pulses. Neither the patients nor the researchers knew which group was receiving the real treatment.

The results were intriguing: By the end of the experimental period, twenty-nine of the thirty men in the ETG group had regrown hair or halted further hair loss. After counting a designated square inch on each man's scalp, the researchers found that the extent of regrowth was 66 percent more hair. No one experienced any side effects or unusual reactions, either.

Two years later, the same researchers conducted another study involving thirty-four of the original participants. Those who had received the placebo treatment in the previous study were

offered ETG—and grew new hair in the process. Other participants enhanced their hair growth. On average, the number of terminal (normal) hairs in those people receiving ETG treatment
increased from 82 to 276.

A larger clinical trial followed later, conducted at test centers
across the United States and Canada, and involved three hundred
men and three hundred women. Again, there were positive
results in both men and women.

How ETG Works

Although these are the results of just three studies to date, they
seem to show that ETG works. But how?

The Canadian researchers believe that the electrical pulses
may increase cell division in the follicle and dermal papilla cells,
thus regenerating dormant hair follicles. ETG, however, does not
work on hair follicles that have already died. What's more, the
treatment works best if you've just begun to experience hair loss,
not if you've been balding for a long time. ETG seems to stop hair
loss better than it regrows hair.

As with any hair-loss treatment, results vary from person to
person. Some people may notice decreased shedding as early as
four to six weeks. With others, it may take longer. Also, if you quit
treatment, any new hair you have grown is likely to fall out, and
shedding will resume, according to Current Technology.

Clearly, ETG offers some benefit. The problem is that a lot of
other companies are jumping on the bandwagon and selling electrical hair stimulation devices, some for home use, that have not
been scientifically tested. These products probably will not give
the same results as the ETG treatment developed by Current
Technology.

For more information on ETG and Current Technology Corporation, contact the company at 1250–800 West Pender Street,
Vancouver, British Columbia, V6C 2V6 Canada; 604–684-2727
or toll-free in the United States and Canada, 800–661-4247;
www.currentech.com.

PART 4

You Hair
What
You Eat

EIGHT

All-Around Best Diet to Support Hair Regrowth

C AN YOU eat your way to a better head of hair?

Not exactly. Although the health of your hair does reflect the quality of your diet, there's no sound nutritional evidence that eating certain foods will restore hair growth. It's best to follow a balanced diet that includes a variety of foods from all the important food groups and that does not skimp on important nutrients.

On the other hand, poor nutrition can cause hair loss. In response to a low intake of protein, vitamins, or minerals, your body rations out stored nutrients in a hierarchy. Your vital organs are nourished first, and your hair last, simply because your brain considers the hair as less essential.

Thus, by improving your diet, you may be able to minimize the shedding. Further, good nutrition can enhance medical treatments that promote hair regrowth—and make your new and existing hair healthier and more radiant than ever before. Here's a look at the major nutrients that make up a hair-healthy diet.

Protein

Your body is constructed entirely of protein. Of all nutrients, protein is perhaps the most important because it is found in every cell. In fact, the word *protein* comes from a Greek word meaning "first." There are different kinds of protein in your body, too. One of these is keratin, the protein found in hair and nails.

When you wash your face, whole cells are sloughed off from the surface of your skin. After you cut your hair or fingernails, new growth occurs. Similarly, other cells of the body, which die or are lost through normal physiological processes, must constantly be replaced. Protein from food is required to build new cells to replace those that are lost.

The protein you eat is broken down into fragments called amino acids. These are used to construct new body tissues, including hair; enzymes and hormones, which regulate all body processes; and antibodies, which fight off infection and disease. At the cellular level, amino acids form DNA and RNA, special proteins inside cells that control cellular growth and reproduction.

Numbering twenty-two in all, amino acids are divided into two groups: essential, or indispensable, amino acids; and dispensable, or nonessential, amino acids. Essential amino acids cannot be manufactured by the body, or are manufactured in very small amounts. You must get them from protein foods and combinations of vegetable foods.

Your body continually takes apart amino acids in foods and then uses them to create new protein—in your blood, in your hair and fingernails, and in your muscles. In fact, your body cannot manufacture protein unless all of the essential amino acids are present. There are nine essential amino acids: histidine, isoleucine, leucine, lysine, methionine, phenylalanine, threonine, tryptophan, and valine.

As for nonessential amino acids, your body can manufacture them from vitamins and other amino acids. The term *nonessential* is somewhat of a misnomer though, since all amino acids are vital to good health. Plus, nonessential amino acids become very essential during sickness and stress. The thirteen nonessential amino acids are alanine, arginine, asparagine, aspartic acid, cysteine, cystine, glutamic acid, glutamine, glycine, hydroxyproline, proline, serine, and tyrosine.

Four amino acids are directly involved in hair growth: cystine, cysteine, methionine, and arginine. Supplementation with these amino acids is often recommended in the treatment of hair loss.

Another amino implicated in hair loss is lysine, which is essential for the formation of collagen, the repair of tissue, and the absorption of calcium, among other functions. If you're deficient in lysine, your hair can fall out.

In addition, lysine is one of the protein particles bonded to copper in various topical lotions used to treat hair loss. This bonded blend is called a "copper peptide," and it appears to help promote cell division in the hair matrix. Lysine is found mostly in lean meats, fish, potatoes, and milk. For more information on amino acid supplementation, see Chapter Eleven.

To support hair growth and health, an adequate amount of protein-rich foods should be a part of your daily diet. If you shun protein, or embark on a crash diet, your body will start to conserve protein as a defense mechanism by shifting growing hairs into a resting phase. The follicles will begin to cast off hair a few months later. But you can reverse this situation by populating your diet with more protein.

Excellent sources of protein include lean meats, poultry, fish, eggs, dairy products, soy foods, legumes, grains, nuts, and seeds.

Carbohydrates

Carbohydrates are energy foods. They provide the fuel for activity and for the growth of all body tissues, including hair growth. Cereals, pasta, breads, fruits, and vegetables are all examples of carbohydrates.

Carbohydrates are a chief source of B-complex vitamins, nutrients that are vital to healthy hair. Modern diets are often deficient in B-complex vitamins simply because we eat too many overly refined carbohydrates, namely sugar, white flour, and breads. The refining process strips away many vital nutrients, including B-complex vitamins. A hair-healthy diet should include natural, nonrefined carbohydrates such as whole grains and cereals, brown rice, legumes, potatoes, yams, fruits, and vegetables.

Dietary Fats

For your hair to be healthy and lustrous, you need some fat in your diet. Fat is a nutrient involved mostly in energy production. Found in both animal and plant foods, fats are chemically classified into three groups according to their hydrogen content: saturated, polyunsaturated, and monounsaturated.

Saturated fats are usually solid at room temperature and, with the exception of tropical oils, come from animal sources. Beef fat and butterfat are high in saturated fats, while low-fat or skimmed milk products are much lower in saturated fat. Tropical oils high in saturated fat include coconut oil, palm kernel oil, and palm oil, and the cocoa fat found in chocolate. They are generally found in commercial baked goods and other processed foods.

Polyunsaturated and monounsaturated fats are usually liquid at room temperature and come from nut, vegetable, or seed sources. Monounsaturated fats are found in large amounts in olive oil, canola oil, and peanut oil, and in fish from cold waters, such as salmon, mackerel, halibut, swordfish, black cod, and rainbow trout, and in shellfish.

There's a lot of talk about cutting fat in the diet. But if you slash fat to miniscule levels, or cut it out altogether, you risk an essential fat deficiency. One of the side effects is hair loss.

On the other hand, too much fat in your diet can also spell trouble, ultimately leading to an overproduction of testosterone and other androgens. Here's how this happens: A diet high in animal fat causes your system to churn out too much cholesterol, an odorless, waxy fatlike substance found in all animal foods but made naturally by the human body. Cholesterol is a building block of testosterone. But an excess of cholesterol (triggered by a high-fat diet) leads to higher-than-normal concentrations of testosterone and other androgens.

Proof of this first surfaced recently when researchers at the Inaba Hair Institute in Tokyo sought an explanation for the dramatic increase in hair loss among Japanese men in the period following World War II. The common denominator was diet. An analysis of postwar diets revealed that the Japanese diet had become "Westernized"; the men were eating an excess of foods high in animal fats, which had elevated cholesterol levels in their bodies. Their dietary lifestyle was making them go bald!

In addition, a high-fat diet reduces levels of a protein called *sex hormone binding globulin*. This protein keeps sex hormones under wraps until needed by the body. When it is in short supply, testosterone is free to circulate in the body, and is vulnerable to being converted to DHT.

At the hair follicle, sebaceous glands contain 5 alpha-reductase, the enzyme that morphs testosterone into DHT. Higher levels of testosterone bathing the hair follicle can increase the production of DHT. Thus, a high-fat diet wreaks hormonal havoc in the body.

So where's the happy medium—between too much fat and too little? Exactly how much fat should you eat daily for normalized hormone levels and good health?

Technically, the maximum amount of fat considered healthy in your daily diet is 30 percent or less, based on the number of calories you eat. Saturated fat should be 10 percent or less of total daily calories; monounsaturated and polyunsaturated fats should also be at 10 percent or less.

If you don't have a head for math and hate counting grams, simply populate your diet with plenty of natural foods. Fill up on whole-grain breads, cereals, legumes, vegetables, and fruits, and eat smaller portions of meats. This approach is similar to a vegetarian way of eating. Studies show that vegetarians have lower levels of testosterone in their blood.

Planning a Hair-Healthy Diet

To support hair growth and health, plan your diet with most of your calories from grain products, vegetables, fruits, low-fat milk products, lean meats, fish, poultry, and dry beans. Choose fewer calories from fats and sweets. High-sugar diets deplete your body of vitamins and minerals.

Make sure to eat a variety of foods, too. Foods contain combinations of nutrients and other healthful substances. No single food can supply all nutrients in the amounts you need.

The U.S. Department of Agriculture has created excellent dietary guidelines for Americans, and these guidelines help ensure that you obtain maximum nutrition from your meals. Here's how you can plan your meals according to the food groups established by the Department of Agriculture.

FOOD CHOICES AND SERVING SIZES

Bread, Cereal, Rice, and Pasta
(6–11 servings)
1 serving = 1 slice of bread; 1 ounce of ready-to-eat cereal;
1/2 cup of cooked cereal, rice, or pasta

Vegetables
(3-5 servings)
Vegetables are loaded with health-building nutrients. Try to eat a variety of vegetables in a variety of colors. Choose dark, green leafy vegetables, deep-yellow or orange vegetables, and starchy vegetables such as potatoes, sweet potatoes, and yams.

1 serving = 1 cup of raw leafy vegetables; 1/2 cup of other vegetables, cooked or chopped raw; 3/4 cup of vegetable juice

Fruits
(2-3 servings)
Fruits are another food packed with health-building nutrients.

Your best choices are fresh fruits and juices, and frozen or dried fruits.

1 serving = 1 medium apple, banana, orange; 1/2 cup of chopped, cooked, canned, or frozen fruit; 3/4 cup of fruit juice

Milk, Yogurt, and Cheese
(2-3 servings)
Choose low-fat varieties to keep saturated fat in check. Saturated fat found in animal foods is responsible for elevating the bad cholesterol in the body.

1 serving = 1 cup of skim milk, soy milk, or low-fat or nonfat yogurt; 2 ounces of processed low-fat or nonfat cheese, tofu, cottage cheese

Meat, Poultry, Fish, Dry Beans, Eggs, and Nuts and Seeds
(2-3 servings)
Select low-fat varieties of animal proteins such as lean red meat, white meat poultry, and fish.

1 serving = 2-3 ounces of cooked lean meat, poultry, or fish; 1/2 cup of cooked dry beans; 1 egg; 2 egg whites; 2 tablespoons nuts or seeds

Fats, Oils, and Sweets
Choose these foods sparingly.

As you can see, these guidelines provide a range of servings for each food group. The smaller number is for people who consume about 1,600 calories a day, such as many sedentary women. The larger number is for those who consume about 2,800 calories a day and are more active.

Notice, too, that some of the serving sizes are smaller than what you might usually eat. For example, many people eat a cup or more of rice in a meal, which equals two or more servings. So it is easy to eat the number of servings recommended.

Some foods fit into more than one group. Dry beans, peas, and lentils can be counted as servings in either the meat and beans group or vegetable group.

Should You Supplement Your Diet?

If you're following a nutritious diet as outlined above, should you take nutritional supplements such as vitamins and minerals and other supplements if your hair is thinning?

Answer: probably—for several reasons.

To begin with, our foods today are not as nutritious as they once were. Modern farming methods, for example, have depleted the soil in many areas of the country, ultimately diminishing the nutrient quality of food. Also, weight-loss diets can increase your need for nutrients. Cooking can destroy certain vitamins, too.

Stress is another factor that depletes the nutrients in your body. Suppose you are stuck in traffic, it is 2:30 P.M., and you're late for an important meeting. The entire time, your body is rapidly using up vitamin C and the B vitamins. That single stressful situation has just predisposed you to a nutrient-deficient state. Under unresolved stressful conditions, your adrenal glands start churning out extra androgens (including testosterone) and they stay dangerously elevated in your body.

Further, many people do not eat nutritiously enough to even satisfy the recommended dietary allowances (RDA) for vitamins, minerals, and other nutrients, according to research. Numerous studies have shown that a majority of the population does not consume enough protein, calcium, iron, magnesium, vitamin A, B-complex vitamins, and vitamin C for good health.

No two women are alike in their need for various nutrients, either. Our own individual nutrient requirements vary, depending on age, activity level, and overall physical health.

With age, for example, your need for certain nutrients change. People over sixty, for example, have trouble absorbing enough

Wilma F. Bergfeld, M.D., F.A.C.P.
1992 President of the American Academy of Dermatology
Head of Dermatology, Clinical Research, and Dermatopathology at the Cleveland Clinic

Dr. Bergfeld is a leading authority on hair loss and androgen disorders. She believes that nutrition plays an important supportive role in treating women's hair loss.

"Nutritional therapy includes rational dieting such as the American Heart Association diet or the Weight Watchers low-fat diet with low sodium (salt)," she says. "An excessive weight gain of twenty or more pounds in short periods of time is frequently accompanied by hair loss. This is thought to be secondary to dietary and mineral deficiencies.

"A one-a-day multiple vitamin and mineral supplement with added folic acid and biotin is clinically helpful. Of course, iron supplementation may be key, too. Women who are vegetarians may not be consuming enough absorbable iron, and women who are still menstruating may need additional iron, too."

folic acid (a B vitamin), vitamin B_{12}, and calcium. Age also ups our need for iron and silica—two hair-healthy minerals.

Exercise depletes some nutrients, particularly minerals. Thus, if you're physically active, you may benefit from additional nutrients. Taking extra doses of antioxidants—namely vitamins E and C—has been found in studies to be very useful.

Supplementation is thus an excellent way to guard against health-damaging deficiencies. Supplements, however, are not a cure for baldness or thinning hair, unless your hair loss is caused by a nutritional deficiency. Rather, they are a supportive, complementary treatment—one that helps create an environment for optimal hair growth and health.

Thus, a good motto to adopt is: Food first; supplements, second. Before you even consider taking supplements, make sure you're following a nutritious diet, as outlined in the previous chapter. Only then should you add supplements to your diet.

In the next five chapters, we'll take a closer look at the specific vitamins, minerals, amino acids, herbs, and other nutritional supplements you can take to enhance the health of your hair.

NINE

Vitamins for Healthy Hair

V ITAMINS are nutrients found in food that assist in the growth of all body tissues and help release energy in the body. Your body cannot make vitamins. You have to get them from food—the best source—and from nutritional supplements as a backup.

There are two classifications of vitamins: water-soluble and fat-soluble. The body cannot store water-soluble vitamins such as the B-complex vitamins and vitamin C because they do not easily penetrate the fat-based membranes of cells. Therefore, they must constantly be replenished by the diet.

Fat-soluble vitamins such as A, D, and E have numerous duties in the body. Unlike water-soluble vitamins, they can enter cell membranes and are thus easily stored in body tissues.

Of the thirteen vitamins necessary for good health, several are involved specifically in hair growth and maintenance. The vitamins your hair needs for good health are summarized in Table 9-1 on page 138.

Table 9-1. Vitamins for Healthy Hair

NUTRIENT	ROLE IN HAIR HEALTH	BEST FOOD SOURCES	DAILY REQUIREMENT
Vitamin A	Enhances health of sebaceous glands in the skin and scalp	Liver, egg yolks, whole milk, and orange and yellow vegetables	5,000 IUs
Vitamin C	Maintains skin collagen and protects hair from undue breakage	Tomatoes, citrus fruits, strawberries, green peppers, potatoes, and dark green vegetables	60 mg
Vitamin E	Enhances scalp circulation and hair quality	Vegetable oils, whole-grain cereals, dried beans, and green, leafy vegetables	Up to 400 IUs
Biotin	May prevent grayness and balding, involved in the production of keratin	Milk, liver, egg yolk, whole grains, rice, and brewer's yeast	150–300 mcg
Inositol	Protects health of hair follicles	Whole grains, citrus fruits, brewer's yeast, and liver	None established
Niacin	Enhances scalp circulation and normalizes cholesterol levels	Chicken, turkey, and fish	15 mg
Vitamin B_5 (Pantothenic acid)	Helps regulate hormones involved in skin and hair health	Organ meats, brewer's yeast, egg yolks, and whole grains	5–7 mg
Vitamin B_6 (Pyroxidine)	With zinc, blocks the conversion of testosterone into DHT	Organ meats, brewer's yeast, egg yolks, and whole grains	1.6 mg
Vitamin B_{12} (Cobalamin)	Can be depleted by CPA therapy	Poultry, fish, eggs, and milk	2 mcg

Vitamin A

Vitamin A is a versatile nutrient because it regulates so many essential functions in the body, including immunity. Compromised immunity is implicated in the alopecia areata type of baldness.

Vitamin A helps fight viral and bacterial infections (also culprits in some types of hair loss), possibly by stimulating the activity of white blood cells. Vitamin A also helps tissues heal faster and keeps the skin healthy. Because your hair is an extension of your skin, this nutrient is vital to hair health. It helps the sebaceous glands in your skin and scalp function normally. A short supply of vitamin A leads to a flaky scalp.

Too much vitamin A, however, can cause your hair to fall out. In large doses (higher than 50,000 IUs daily), vitamin A is toxic because it accumulates in the liver and other organs. The recommended daily intake for vitamin A is 5,000 international units.

Foods rich in vitamin A include liver, egg yolks, whole milk, carrots, all yellow and orange vegetables, and green, leafy vegetables.

B-Complex Vitamins

Vital for energy, the B-complex vitamins are involved in nearly every reaction in the body, from the manufacture of new red blood cells to the metabolism of carbohydrates, fat, and protein. Several members of this family are hair-friendly nutrients. For example:

BIOTIN

Dubbed the "hair vitamin," biotin helps produce healthy hair and may even prevent grayness and balding. It also helps your body utilize protein and is involved in the production of keratin, the protein in hair and nails. If your fingernails are brittle, biotin may be just the remedy you need. Research shows that supplementing with biotin thickens fingernails and keeps their outer layers from peeling off. Biotin's benefit to nails is the reason you find the vitamin in beauty products sold at the cosmetics counter.

Biotin cures an unusual condition called "uncombable hair syndrome," in which hair cannot be combed flat. Taking oral supplements of biotin clears this condition up, often within several months.

Without enough biotin in your diet, you can go bald. Severe hair loss has been observed in tube-fed patients who took in no biotin. But when the patients were given supplemental biotin, their hair came back.

Biotin supports the growth of healthy hair, but may not directly promote hair regrowth. In a study conducted by a group of Polish researchers, twenty-eight women with hair loss took 10 milligrams of biotin daily for twenty-eight days. A control group that included eighteen women received a placebo. By the end of the experimental period, none of the women in either group had experienced any new hair growth.

More research into the biotin–hair regrowth issue, however, is needed. Some alternative health care practitioners report good results with biotin supplementation and often recommend high doses of biotin for short periods of time to reactivate hair growth.

Although required in tiny amounts (150 to 300 micrograms daily), biotin can be in short supply—for one simple reason. The best sources of biotin in food are egg yolks and liver—two foods we tend to eliminate from our diet because of their high concentration of cholesterol.

Even so, such deficiencies are rare, and one reason is that biotin can be manufactured by bacteria in the intestines. It is also distributed in small amounts in foods such as milk, whole grains, and soy flour. Other foods rich in biotin include rice and brewer's yeast.

A dietary practice that interferes with the body's use of biotin is eating raw eggs (which also puts you at risk of contracting salmonella poisoning). Raw egg whites contain a protein called avidin that binds with biotin and keeps it from being absorbed. Cooking eggs inactivates avidin.

Years ago it was believed that people who ate little or no animal products would be at risk for deficiencies. But a fascinating study proved otherwise. A group of researchers compared biotin levels in vegans (people who eat no animal products), lactovegetarians (people who eat eggs and dairy products), and people who eat a normal mixed diet. The researchers had logically assumed that biotin levels would be low in vegans and higher in the other groups. But they were surprised to learn that vegans had the highest levels. Two possible explanations were offered. First, the form of biotin found in plant foods may be the most easily absorbed. Second, vegetarian diets may do a better job at helping intestinal bacteria manufacture ample biotin. If you're a vegetarian, you probably don't need to worry about your biotin intake.

Some nutritional supplements marketed for hair health contain six hundred times the recommended intake of biotin. Carefully read the labels of any biotin-containing supplement.

INOSITOL

This member of the B-complex vitamin family is vital to hair health. Research has found that a short supply of inositol may result in hair loss. In addition, inositol is a white knight of sorts to the hair follicles, protecting them from cellular damage. Deficiencies of inositol have been associated with hair loss.

In the body, inositol combines with another B vitamin, choline, to make lecithin, a fat found in cells and nerve membranes and in egg yolk, soybeans, and corn. Lecithin helps process cholesterol in the body and keeps it from building up in the arteries.

You also need inositol for the normal functioning of your body's cells. It is required by cells in the bone marrow, eye membranes, and intestines for proper growth.

Your body can make inositol from glucose (blood sugar), and the nutrient is plentiful in whole grains. In fact, there is more inositol in the body than any other vitamin, with the exception of the B-vitamin niacin. Too much coffee can deplete your body's reservoir of inositol. This nutrient is available from whole grains, citrus fruits, brewer's yeast, and liver. Each day, you get about a gram of inositol from food.

NIACIN

This member of the B-complex family is found in many nondrug topical formulas designed to treat hair problems. One main reason is that it helps improve circulation throughout the body, including the scalp.

Niacin also helps normalize cholesterol levels in the body. As I have noted earlier, an excess of cholesterol can cause the body to churn out too much testosterone, so it's important to keep this blood fat within healthy levels.

Niacin is also involved in the metabolism of carbohydrates, fats, and protein and is essential for the health of the skin, nervous system, and digestive system. Lean proteins such as chicken, turkey, and fish are excellent sources of niacin. Deficiency symptoms include skin eruptions, fatigue, muscular weakness, and indigestion. For women, the recommended daily intake for niacin is 15 milligrams.

PANTOTHENIC ACID

When a rat's fur turns gray and falls out, it's not due to old age but rather to a pantothenic acid deficiency. Pantothenic acid, sometimes called vitamin B_5, helps regulate hormones that are involved in maintaining healthy skin and hair.

The name pantothenic acid comes from the Greek word *pantothen*, which means "everywhere"—an apt derivative, since this B-complex vitamin is present in every living cell. First recognized as a substance that stimulates growth, pantothenic acid is quite active in metabolism. It is a building block of a key enzyme involved in releasing energy from foods. In addition, pantothenic acid helps the body utilize protein, a major constituent of hair.

Supplementing with pantothenic acid won't promote hair regrowth unless you're deficient in this nutrient. But since it is so widespread in foods, deficiencies are usually not a problem. In addition, the vitamin can be made in the body by intestinal bacteria.

Many multivitamin supplements also contain pantothenic acid. The recommended intake for adults is 4 to 7 milligrams daily. Foods rich in pantothenic acid include organ meats, brewer's yeast, egg yolks, and whole grains.

Known cosmetically as panthenol, pantothenic acid is an ingredient in many hair care products. It moisturizes hair, repairs split ends, and penetrates the hair shaft to give hair a thicker, more vibrant look.

VITAMIN B$_6$ (PYROXIDINE)

This B-complex vitamin influences nearly every system in the body. For example, it assists in metabolizing fats, creating amino acids, turning carbohydrates into usable energy, and manufacturing antibodies to ward off infection.

A few studies have demonstrated that supplemental vitamin B$_6$, when combined with the mineral zinc, can block the conversion of testosterone into DHT in the skin. Other studies show that cells deficient in B$_6$ become overly responsive to hormones such as testosterone. In the case of hair, this means that follicles might be more prone to damage from DHT. However, B$_6$ has not been specifically tested for its effect on hair loss.

The recommended daily intake for vitamin B$_6$ is 1.6 milligrams—roughly the amount found in the average multivitamin pill. Single supplements of vitamin B$_6$ may contain as many as 100 milligrams.

High doses of vitamin B$_6$ can be dangerous. Years ago it was reported that women taking more than 2 grams daily for two months or more for premenstrual syndrome (PMS) symptoms experienced worrisome health problems, including numbness in their feet and loss of sensation in their hands. The problems subsided when the women stopped taking the supplements. The message here: Always read supplement labels, calculate how much of certain nutrients you are taking in, and never megadose.

The best food sources of vitamin B_6 include salmon, Atlantic mackerel, white meat chicken, halibut, tuna, broccoli, lentils, and brown rice.

B_{12} (COBALAMIN)

This nutrient regulates many functions in the body, among the most vital of which is the production of red blood cells. Vitamin B_{12} is the director in this process, making sure that enough cells are manufactured. Without vitamin B_{12}, red blood cell production falls off, and the result is misshapen cells and anemia.

It is not clear exactly what role vitamin B_{12} plays in hair growth. However, we do know that levels of this nutrient are adversely affected by therapy with cyproterone acetate (CPA), taken in conjunction with ethinyl estradiol. These medications are often prescribed in Europe for women suffering hair loss. Women being treated with CPA and ethinyl estradiol should take supplemental vitamin B_{12} (for information on CPA, see pages 52–54).

For most people, though, deficiencies of vitamin B_{12} are rare, as long as a protein-rich diet is followed. The recommended daily intake for vitamin B_{12} is 2 micrograms. This nutrient can be obtained only from animal foods, including poultry, fish, eggs, and milk. Strict vegans (people who eat no food of animal origin), however, are candidates for a B_{12} deficiency.

A serious consequence of vitamin B_{12} deficiency can be irreversible damage to the nervous system. This is because vitamin B_{12} helps build myelin, a protein sheath that envelops your nerves. Nerve tissue degenerates without myelin, causing a host of problems that include numbness, prickly sensations, depression, and memory loss.

Vitamin C

Vitamin C maintains collagen, helps create red blood cells, promotes wound healing, and fights bacterial infection, among other duties. If your hair isn't getting enough vitamin C, it will split and break off more easily.

You need 60 milligrams daily of vitamin C for good health. It is plentiful in tomatoes, citrus fruits, strawberries, green peppers, potatoes, and dark green vegetables.

Vitamin E

Vitamin E is highly recommended by alternative health care practitioners as a must-have nutrient for healthy hair. It enhances circulation to the scalp, thereby improving the delivery of nutrients to the hair follicles. Hair loss and brittle hair may be symptoms of a vitamin E deficiency.

Vitamin E is an antioxidant, meaning that it protects cells from damage, and is thus an important immune-booster. It also interrupts the plaque-forming process that can clog your arteries.

Vitamin E occurs naturally in vegetable oils, whole grain cereals, dried beans, and green, leafy vegetables—yet the content is not high. It's difficult to obtain enough vitamin E from foods to derive the nutrient's many health benefits. Consequently, many nutritionists feel that vitamin E supplements are more effective than food as a means of getting adequate quantities.

Supplementing with 400 international units of vitamin E daily is an excellent way to get the protective amount.

Also, choose a natural form of vitamin E over a synthetic version. Labeled as d-alpha tocopherol, natural vitamin E is isolated from soybean, sunflower, corn, peanut, grapeseed, and cottonseed oils. Synthetic vitamin E, or dl-alpha tocopherol, is processed from substances found in petrochemicals. A recent review of thirty published studies on vitamin E concluded that the natural version is absorbed better by the body than the synthetic form.

TEN

Hair-Building Minerals

MINERALS are important for the formation of bones and tissue and are involved in many physiological processes, including metabolism and energy production. The following minerals are hair-healthy nutrients that are required for proper hair growth and maintenance. Their role in hair health is summarized in Table 10-1 on page 147.

Boron

Found in tomatoes, green peppers, and other vegetables, this trace mineral has great importance in nutrition, especially in mineral metabolism. It helps your body process, handle, and absorb other vital minerals, including calcium, phosphorus, and magnesium. Boron is needed in small amounts for healthy bones and tissue. Because of its supporting role in mineral metabolism, it is often found in nutritional supplements marketed for hair health. However, most people get enough boron without supplementing.

Personal-care products, from shampoos to lipsticks, also contain boron.

Calcium

Of all minerals in the body, calcium is the most abundant. About 99 percent of the calcium in your body is deposited in bones and teeth; the remaining percent is concentrated in the soft tissues.

Table 10-1. Minerals for Healthy Hair

NUTRIENT	ROLE IN HAIR HEALTH	BEST FOOD SOURCES	DAILY REQUIREMENT
Boron	Helps the body metabolize other minerals	Tomatoes, green peppers, and other vegetables	None established
Calcium	A structural component of hair	Dairy products, kale, turnip greens, and broccoli	1,200 mg; 1,500 mg in postmenopausal women
Copper	Involved in normal hair growth; helps prevent defects in the color and structure of hair	Shellfish, liver, cherries, whole grains, eggs, poultry, and beans	1.5–3 mg
Iodine	Helps produce thyroid hormones, which nourish follicles and sebaceous glands	Iodized salt, milk, seaweed products	150 mcg
Iron	Involved in hair growth and maintenance	Lean red meats, dark meat of chicken and turkey; liver; green, leafy vegetables; dried fruits; and iron-enriched foods	15 mg
Magnesium	Helps the body metabolize other minerals	Chickpeas, beet greens, and turnip greens	280 mg
Manganese	Assists the body in using other hair-healthy nutrients	Whole grains, egg yolks, and green vegetables	3–9 mg
Selenium	Preserves skin elasticity	Bran, tuna, broccoli, and onions	55 mcg
Silica	Enhances strength and health of hair	Alfalfa; beets; brown rice; bell peppers; soybeans; green, leafy vegetables; and whole grains	None established
Sulfur	A constituent of hair	Meat, fish, legumes, nuts, eggs, and cabbage	None established
Zinc	With vitamin B_6, blocks the conversion of testosterone into DHT	Red meat, oysters, nuts, seeds, whole grains, and brewer's yeast	12 mg

Calcium is an important structural component of all body tissues, including hair.

Dairy products are the best known of the calcium-rich foods, with a cup of skim milk supplying about 290 milligrams. Vegetables are high in calcium as well, and some of the best sources are kale, turnip greens, and broccoli. Another excellent source is canned salmon with bones.

Calcium needs vary. You need 1,200 milligrams daily; 1,500 milligrams if you are postmenopausal.

Copper

Found in all body tissues, copper is a busy mineral. It assists in bone and collagen formation, energy metabolism, nerve transmission, and red cell production. In addition, copper is involved in normal hair growth and helps prevent defects in the color and structure of hair. Among the signs of copper deficiency is baldness.

Most of the copper in your body is stored in your liver. However, significant amounts are also found in skin, brain, bone marrow, bone, and muscle.

For good health, you need between 1.5 and 3 milligrams of copper a day. By eating a well-balanced diet with a variety of wholesome foods, you should take in plenty of copper. Diets high in sugar, however, tend to be low in copper.

Copper is present in nutritionally significant amounts in nearly all foods. It is particularly abundant in shellfish, liver, cherries, whole grains, eggs, poultry, and beans.

Iodine

Although distributed throughout the body, iodine is concentrated mostly in the thyroid gland, a triangular piece of tissue surrounding the front of the esophagus and windpipe. Iodine's only duty is in the formation of two thyroid hormones. One of these is thyroxin, which is required by the hair follicles and sebaceous glands for proper functioning. Thyroxin helps nourish these hair structures.

Iodine deficiencies can show up as premature gray hair, dull hair, and loss of hair.

Deficiencies are rarely a problem in Westernized nations, however, since iodine is purposely added to table salt. Sea vegetables such as kelp are the most naturally rich sources of iodine.

Some alternative health practitioners recommend kelp supplementation to promote healthy hair. But you have to be careful not to get too much of a good thing. The recommended daily intake for iodine is 150 micrograms, which you can easily obtain by drinking a cup of milk or salting your food with less than half a teaspoon of iodized salt. At levels of more than 2,000 micrograms—an amount only a few times higher than the amount we get daily—iodine can be toxic. It can cause an enlarged thyroid gland and disrupt the normal functioning of thyroid hormones. If you are considering kelp supplements, be sure to note how much iodine you're already getting from other sources. And, before supplementing, discuss the use of kelp with your physician.

Iron

Iron is vital for growth of all body tissues and for a healthy immune system. In addition, it's absolutely critical to support hair regrowth. If you're losing your hair for no apparent reason, you may be suffering from an iron deficiency. Brittle hair is another sign that iron may be in short supply. Nearly half a million people in the United States and 500 million globally are at risk for this condition. Those in the high-risk category include:

- Women of childbearing age who have heavy periods. Iron gets flushed out with the blood flow.
- Women who have just given birth. Breastfeeding infants use up a lot of the mother's iron stores.
- Vegans—strict vegetarians who eat no meat or dairy products.
- Anyone who consumes a nutrient-poor diet.

A blood test will reveal whether you are iron-needy. Iron status is assessed by measuring ferritin, an iron-storing protein that is present in every cell. A healthy concentration of ferritin is a reading of above forty.

If you're low in iron, your physician may recommend supplementation to correct the problem. But unless a specific deficiency is detected, you don't need to take iron supplements. Taking iron pills unnecessarily has been known to cause telogen effluvium.

Instead, include iron-rich foods in your diet. These include lean red meats and the dark meat of chicken and turkey. Certain fruits, vegetables, and grains are also high in iron: green, leafy vegetables like kale and collards, dried fruits like raisins and apricots, and iron-enriched and fortified breads and cereals. However, the iron from animal foods is more readily absorbed.

You can enhance your body's absorption of iron by combining high iron-containing foods with a rich source of vitamin C, which helps the body better absorb iron. So drink some orange juice with your iron-fortified cereal with raisins for breakfast. Or sprinkle some lemon juice on your kale or collards.

In addition, moderate exercise, especially when combined with a nutritious diet, helps improve your body's use of iron.

The recommended daily intake for iron is 15 milligrams for women. This is easily obtainable from food. Also, multivitamin/mineral supplements usually contain the recommended levels of iron.

Magnesium

Nutritionists have long known that the typical American diet is low in magnesium, a mineral that's involved in many metabolic functions. It is important to hair health because it assists the body in using other minerals, particularly calcium. In fact, calcium can't be metabolized without magnesium.

Magnesium-rich foods include chickpeas, beet greens, and turnip greens. You need 280 milligrams of magnesium daily for good health.

Manganese

This important trace mineral assists the body in using zinc and biotin (the hair vitamin). It also normalizes the action of hormones—a role that makes manganese a vital member of the supporting cast of hair-healthy nutrients.

Manganese is also involved in the formation of bone and cartilage, and it plays a role in protein, carbohydrate, and fat production. Deficiency symptoms include poor muscular coordination, abnormal brain function, glucose tolerance problems, and poor skeletal and cartilage formation. One cause of manganese deficiency appears to be the overconsumption of simple sugars.

You need 3 to 9 milligrams of manganese daily for good health. Foods loaded with manganese include whole grains, egg yolks, and green vegetables.

Selenium

Selenium is a trace mineral that works with other nutrients to guard against disease and build immunity. This mineral has become best known as an antioxidant because it preserves the elasticity of the skin.

Selenium is found in the bran of cereals, in tuna, and in such vegetables as broccoli and onions. You need at least 55 micrograms a day of selenium. Excessively high selenium intake (more than 200 micrograms daily) may cause hair loss.

Silica

Silica is a trace mineral found in plants. Supplemental silica is derived from extracts of the herb horsetail (see page 164), or from algae. This mineral is involved in the formation of bone and collagen and is essential for healthy nails, skin, and hair.

Though rare, some cases of hair loss have been attributed to a silica deficiency. Supplementing with silica has been known to strengthen hair.

You'll find silica as an ingredient in nutritional supplements promoted as hair-restorers. It also comes in a gel. There is probably no harm in supplementing with silica, and some alternative care practitioners believe it's worth looking into if you want healthier hair.

Foods high in silica include alfalfa, beets, brown rice, bell peppers, soybeans, green leafy vegetables, and whole grains.

Sulfur

Sulfur is found in every cell in your body, but it is concentrated mostly in your hair, skin, and nails. In fact, sulfur has been nicknamed the "beauty mineral" because it keeps hair shiny and healthy. Sulfur is an important constituent of the amino acids cystine and cysteine, both involved in hair health. In addition, sulfur is abundant in keratin, the hair protein.

There's no recommended daily intake for sulfur. If you eat enough protein, you'll consume an ample amount of sulfur. Foods rich in sulfur include meat, fish, legumes, nuts, eggs, cabbage, and Brussels sprouts.

Zinc

Present in every nook and cranny of the body, zinc has an array of functions. Among the most important is promoting the general growth of all body tissues, including hair and skin. Zinc appears to be beneficial in treating both androgenetic alopecia and alopecia areata.

Some physicians who treat hair loss believe that zinc works in partnership with vitamin B_6 to block the production of DHT, the hormone that triggers hair loss. The recommended treatment dosage is 100 milligrams of B_6 and 25 milligrams of zinc gluconate daily. Anecdotally, some people who have supplemented with zinc to minimize hair loss say it does the trick.

In 1976 a study published in a medical book reported that two patients with alopecia areata regrew their hair after taking oral supplements of zinc sulfate. Several years later, a scientist decided to further investigate the effects of zinc sulfate on alopecia areata. In his test, he gave either 220 milligrams of zinc sulfate or a placebo to forty-two volunteers suffering from alopecia areata. None of the volunteers knew if they were receiving the zinc or the placebo. After three months of treatment, no improvement in hair growth occurred. Further investigations into zinc's effect on hair regrowth are needed.

Zinc has numerous jobs in the body. For example, it helps absorb vitamins, break down carbohydrates, synthesize protein in cells, construct collagen in the skin, and boost immunity.

Zinc deficiencies could be on the rise, since our soils are becoming depleted of this mineral. What's more, stress also depletes the body of zinc.

Diets high in protein and whole-grain products are usually loaded with zinc. Among other zinc-endowed foods are red meat, oysters, nuts, seeds, and brewer's yeast.

Normally, you need only 12 milligrams daily of zinc; if breast-feeding, you need 19 milligrams. Most diets supply between 10 and 15 milligrams a day.

Hair Savers: What the Experts Recommend

Philip Kingsley
Consultant Trichologist
Philip Kingsley Trichological Centre

Philip Kingsley is a consultant, writer, researcher, and author, with practices in London and New York City. He is the author of *The Complete Hair Book* (Grosset and Dunlap, 1979) and *Hair: An Owner's Handbook* (Aurum, 1997). In addition, he has researched and coauthored two major scientific studies on women's hair loss, published in the *Journal of the American Academy of Dermatology* and *Clinical and Experimental Dermatology*, respectively.

(continued on page 154)

(continued from page 153)

For women with androgenetic alopecia, Mr. Kingsley recommends the following:

• Have a blood test to check iron levels, including ferritin; nutritional status; and androgens. On blood tests, normal ferritin levels can start as low as 15, and a reading of 30 is well within the normal range. However, research shows that a ferritin level below 70 could cause hair problems.

• Use 150 to 200 milligrams of spironolactone, taken orally and/or as a topical antiandrogen. Spironolactone is available only through a physician.

• Eat protein at each meal.

For alopecia areata, Mr. Kingsley explains that this condition usually reverses itself spontaneously. "In the two percent or so of cases that do not, the application of a strong counterirritant and ultraviolet radiation, or cortisone, can be effective.

"Take good cosmetic care of the hair by shampooing and conditioning daily; and using whatever styling aid is necessary," he adds. "The psychological effect of good-looking hair is considerable."

ELEVEN

Protein Powerhouse: Amino Acid Supplements

AMINO ACIDS are the natural building blocks of dietary protein and found in nearly all foods. They are also sold as supplements. Available as capsules, tablets, liquids, and powders, amino acid supplements are made from animal protein, yeast protein, or vegetable protein.

Individual amino acids are used therapeutically to treat certain health conditions, including hair loss and shedding. As I noted earlier, the following amino acids are often recommended for treating hair loss:

Arginine

Arginine is considered a nonessential amino acid, meaning the body can synthesize it from proteins and other nutrients. Despite the fact that arginine is labeled nonessential, it has a number of important functions in the body. For example, it helps release growth hormone to support growth, including hair growth. Arginine also helps keep the body from breaking down protein in muscles and organs to repair itself when injured.

Arginine is highly concentrated in the skin and connective tissues, where it helps heal and repair damaged tissue.

According to anecdotal reports, some balding men have taken arginine in combination with saw palmetto and *pygeum africanum*—with good results. (For information on herbs and hair loss, see Chapter Twelve.)

Although an important nutrient for growth, supplemental arginine has not yet been scientifically tested for its role in preventing and treating hair loss.

Foods rich in arginine include brown rice, nuts, seeds, oatmeal, cereals, raisins, and whole-wheat products.

If you supplement with arginine, follow the manufacturer's dosage recommendation. Also, don't supplement with arginine for longer than several weeks. It may thicken your skin and roughen its texture, especially if dosages are excessive.

Don't take supplemental arginine if you have herpes or schizophrenia; it can aggravate these conditions. Pregnant and lactating women should also avoid supplemental arginine.

Cysteine and Cystine

These amino acids are chemical cousins. Each molecule of cystine is constructed of two molecules of cysteine intertwined together, and either amino acid can convert to the other if needed by the body. In addition, both are sulfur-containing amino acids involved in the formation of skin and hair.

Cysteine assists in the production of collagen and gives your skin greater elasticity. It also destroys disease-causing free radicals and works best at this job when taken in conjunction with selenium and vitamin E.

Cystine has other duties in the body. It boosts levels of glutathione, a powerful antioxidant enzyme that detoxifies carcinogens and has the power to turn free radicals into water. Because of its many health-boosting talents, cystine is also considered to be an antiaging nutrient.

Keratin (the hair protein) is rich in both cystine and cysteine. Supplied by a protein-rich diet or by supplements, both nutrients can improve the quality, texture, and growth of your hair. They may even help minimize fall-out.

Cystine, in particular, has some scientific backing to support its role in treating hair loss. In two 1989 studies, a group of German researchers gave 70 milligrams of cystine, 18,000 international units of retinol (a vitamin A derivative), and 700 milligrams of gelatin to patients suffering from hair loss. Other patients received a placebo. In both studies, the hair-growing cycle increased (by 11 percent in the first study and by 8 percent in the second). Also, hair density, measured in the first study, increased by nearly 7 percent. There were no changes in the placebo group. The researchers concluded that "long-term oral therapy with high doses of l-cystine and gelatin in combination with vitamin A may have beneficial effects on diffuse hair loss."

Worth noting, however, is that it's hard to pinpoint in this study which nutrient conferred the biggest benefit. Perhaps they worked synergistically as a team.

Because cysteine is more soluble than cystine, it's absorbed and used more easily by the body. The recommended dosage for treating hair loss is 500 milligrams twice a day on an empty stomach. You can take cysteine with water or juice.

If you have diabetes, do not supplement with cysteine; it can inactivate insulin.

Lysine

Lysine is an essential amino acid that aids in the absorption of calcium from food and is involved in the formation of the matrix of bone, cartilage, and connective tissue. It helps build muscle as well.

Lysine also acts as an antioxidant that attacks disease-causing free radicals, and in that regard, is a good immune-booster. Lysine is also involved in the cell division that takes in the hair matrix. A deficiency of lysine can lead to hair loss.

Dairy products, fish, meats, lima beans, soy products, and potatoes are all high in lysine. If considering supplementation, follow the manufacturer's dosage guidelines.

Methionine

Your body uses the essential amino acid methionine to form cysteine. Methionine also plays a number of other important roles in the body. It is a mighty antioxidant, a neutralizer of harmful toxins, and a regulator of estrogen.

As for hair, alternative health care practitioners believe that methionine enhances the look and feel of hair and may help prevent it from falling out.

Rich food sources of methionine include eggs, fish, meat, and milk. There is no appreciable amount of methionine in plant foods.

The recommended supplemental dosage of methionine is 500 milligrams twice a day on an empty stomach. You can take methionine with water or juice. In addition, both cysteine and methionine can be taken together.

Supplementing with Amino Acids

Do not take amino acid supplements for long periods of time, because they may cause nutrient imbalances. It's a good idea to take an amino acid supplement in an on-and-off cycle. Supplement for two or three months, stop for two or three months, then resume supplementation, and so forth. And consult your physician before supplementing with amino acids.

TWELVE

Anti-Baldness Herbs

C AN HERBS reverse baldness?
At least one study, conducted with mice, says yes. Several years ago in Japan, a rather amazing animal study revealed that herbs could significantly boost hair growth.

Intrigued by the fact that many herbal extracts are ingredients in hair tonics, a group of scientists investigated eighty different herbs to see which ones stimulated hair growth. They discovered that eighteen herbs, applied topically in a cream base, did the trick. The most potent of the hair-growing herbs were rich in natural fats, long known to help promote hair health.

Of course, there's no proof yet that the mouse experience will translate into the same positive results in humans. Plus, most of the herbs used in the study were rather obscure—not those you would readily find in an American health food store. But the possibilities are fascinating nonetheless. After all, who wouldn't prefer taking a natural remedy, like an herb, that you can get in a health food store or pharmacy to taking a prescription drug?

Although slowly, evidence is surfacing that certain herbs, applied topically or taken orally as pills, may counteract baldness in some cases. Consequently, numerous alternative health care practitioners are recommending that people with thinning and balding hair at least give herbs a try. Many of the nondrug topical formulas described in Chapter Five contain hair-friendly herbs.

This chapter looks at what herbs are, which ones can be taken orally, and which ones are used topically to treat baldness.

What Are Herbs?

An herb is a plant or a part of a plant that is valued for its medicinal qualities, aroma, or taste. Herbs and herbal remedies have been used for healing down through the ages, in every culture and civilization. Until the twentieth century, physicians routinely prescribed herbal-based medicines for their patients. In fact, your grandmother and great-grandmother probably relied on herbs to treat illnesses in their day.

Nearly 50 percent of all modern drugs are derived from herbs or contain a chemical imitation of a plant compound. One of the best known is aspirin. In the early 1800s, its active ingredient, salicin, was isolated from white willow bark, an anti-inflammatory plant used for thousands of years, and eventually synthesized into a chemical imitation, known to us as aspirin. Pencillin, the kingpin of all antibiotics, is a mold produced by a type of primitive plant known as a fungus. Digitalis, an important drug used to treat congestive heart failure, was discovered two hundred years ago from an ingredient in foxglove, a common garden flower grown in England. Quinidine, an important cardiac drug, and its relative quinine, long used to treat malaria, both come from the bark of the Peruvian cinchona tree. Another bark-derived drug, taxol, now shows promise as a powerful cancer-fighting drug. Even today, pharmaceutical companies are scouring rain forests and other primitive locales to find native remedies and botanicals that may hold the cures for modern diseases.

Today, there is a revival of tidal-wave proportions in the use of herbs to treat all kinds of disease. It's estimated that 60 million Americans now take herbs to help cure what ails them, from colds to allergies, from headaches to baldness. And according to the World Health Organization, 80 percent of the world's population uses herbs.

The reason for such popularity is that herbs work with the body's natural healing mechanisms, not against them. Generally, herbs have been found to provide additional nutrients that restore health, protect the immune system, and normalize body functions. Thus, herbal therapy is an effective, natural way to help the body heal itself.

As for treating baldness, some herbs may provide some help. But they are certainly not a cure-all, and I can't promise that your hair will return to its former crowning glory if you take herbs. Worth noting, too, is that the German Commission E, Germany's equivalent to our FDA, makes no recommendations on herbal treatments for baldness in its monographs, a publication that describes scores of herbs and their therapeutic applications.

To help you sort out fact from fiction, here is a look at the numerous herbs being touted for their hair-restoring properties, and the research, if any, behind them—and what they can and cannot do for hair health and baldness.

Oral Herbal Supplements

FO-TI OR HO SHOU WU (POLYGONUM MULTIFLORUM)

Chinese herbalists swear that this member of the buckwheat family works wonders for restoring hair loss and preventing gray hair. In fact, the name *shou-wu* means "a head full of black hair" in Chinese.

In China, many health care professionals believe that if your hair is falling out or turning prematurely gray, there's an imbalance in your kidneys, liver, or blood. Fo-ti, they say, is just the tonic needed to rebalance the system. This improvement will thus show up as healthier hair. While there are many Asian studies confirming certain health benefits to using fo-ti, none specifically proves that the herb will restore hair growth or hair color.

Fo-ti is available as an oral supplement. It's generally considered safe, although there is one case in the medical literature that reports on a thirty-one-year-old woman who contracted hepatitis (a liver disease) after using a Chinese herbal product containing the herb. She was taking the herb to treat hair loss.

GINSENG

Derived from a root, ginseng is a popular herb used to treat numerous ailments, including nervous disorders, anemia, lack of sexual desire, fatigue, and heart problems. There are three types of ginsengs: the Asian variety (*Panax ginseng*); American ginseng (*Panax quinquefolius*); and Siberian ginseng (*Eleutherococcus senticosus*), which originates from a different species than the *Panax* classifications.

Asian ginseng and Siberian ginseng are approved medicines in Germany. In fact, the German Commission E states in its monographs that these ginsengs can be used "as a tonic for invigoration and fortification in times of fatigue and debility, for declining capacity for work and concentration, also during convalescence."

In China today, many preparations of ginseng are officially approved for medicinal use. More than three thousand scientific studies have been conducted on this herb, mainly the Asian variety. In 1998, researchers in South Korea studied the effect of Asian ginseng on the hair follicles of mice that had received doses of radiation. Radiation typically shatters and kills cells, including those in the follicle. Interestingly, ginseng protected against cell destruction in the hair follicle and even seemed to help cells recover. The clinical significance of these findings is not clear, but they hint that ginseng may protect against radiation-induced hair loss.

You find ginseng in teas and as powders, capsules, extracts, tablets, teas, and ginseng-flavored soft drinks. For Asian ginseng, the German Commission E recommends 1 to 2 grams daily of the powdered herb or equivalent for up to three months; for Siberian, 2 to 3 grams of the powdered herb or equivalent for up to three months. Makers of standardized extracts of ginseng generally recommend a daily dose of 200 milligrams.

Side effects of ginseng supplementation are rare, and the herb is considered safe. However, excessive doses and long-term use may cause high blood pressure, nervousness, insomnia, painful breasts, and vaginal bleeding. If you have high blood pressure, avoid ginseng.

GINKGO (*GINGKO BILOBA*)
Gingko biloba, derived from the leaves of an ornamental tree, improves blood circulation to the skin and brain. Increased blood flow helps deliver more nutrients to hair follicles, which is why gingko is often counted among the hair-healthy herbs.

At least one animal study has found that gingko might fight baldness. In an experiment published in 1993, a group of Japanese researchers shaved the fur of laboratory mice and gave them some gingko. The herb promoted hair regrowth. Based on these findings, the scientists suggested that gingko could be used as a hair tonic.

While little is really known about a possible benefit, there are plenty of other research-verified reasons to supplement with gingko. The herb appears to improve short- and long-term memory, reduce ringing in the ears (tinnitus), and alleviate headaches. In addition, it may help people with Alzheimer's disease.

Gingko biloba is listed as an approved herb in the German Commission E Monographs. The recommended daily dosage listed in the monographs is between 120 and 160 milligrams of the dry extract in two or three doses.

GREEN TEA (*CAMELLIA SINESIS*)
Sipping a cup or two of green tea daily may put hair loss on the slow track. Preliminary animal research shows that certain natural chemicals, called "catechins," in green tea inhibit 5 alpha-reductase, the enzyme involved in converting testosterone to follicle-killing DHT. Green tea is richer in catechins than black tea is.

Green tea extract is also an ingredient in some hair care products. It supposedly helps strengthen damaged hair.

Even if drinking tea does not restore your hair, it may enhance your health in other ways. Research into the health benefits of both green and black tea has found that the natural chemicals in tea may protect against periodontal disease, cancer, heart disease, and liver illness.

You can reap the benefits of tea in the conventional way—with a serving of brewed or iced tea—or by popping a pill of green tea extract. One cup of green tea contains roughly 100 milligrams of catechins. Depending on the supplement, a single pill may contain as many health-building chemicals as four cups of brewed green tea. If you choose to supplement, follow the manufacturer's dosage recommendations.

HORSETAIL (EQUISETUM ARVENSE)

A close relative to a tree that grew in dinosaur days, this herb is a rich source of silica, a trace mineral involved in hair health and tissue repair.

Horsetail is believed to help increase circulation to the scalp, so that more nutrients can make their way to the hair follicle.

Herbalists have recommended horsetail to treat a wide range of other conditions, including osteoporosis, bronchitis, kidney problems, and bladder disorders. If you supplement with horsetail, follow the manufacturer's dosage recommendations.

KAVA-KAVA (PIPER METHYSTICUM)

The everyday hassles of life can trigger hair loss. In 1998, researchers at Western Kentucky University looked into the stress levels of twenty-five women who had suffered recent, unexplained hair loss, and compared them to twenty-five women who were not experiencing hair loss. It turned out that twenty-two of the women with hair loss were under high stress, compared to ten women with no hair loss. Based on this finding, the researchers concluded that the odds of losing your hair are eleven times more likely if you are stressed out.

A rather unusual case of stress-related alopecia was reported in 1994 in the *Archives of Dermatology*. A married couple, both in their mid-thirties, sought help from a dermatologist after starting to lose their hair—both at about the same time! Exhaustive tests were performed, and the diagnosis was alopecia areata. As to why the loss of hair occurred simultaneously, the only common denominator was stress. The husband began to lose his hair after experiencing severe anxiety over losing his job, then having to relocate to another job. Likewise, his wife, after being fired from her job and losing her father six months earlier, started balding, too.

Other research has found that stress may trigger trichotillomania (the hair-pulling syndrome). It follows, then, that managing and resolving stress may help prevent or reverse hair loss in some cases. Quite often though, stress management is easier said than done.

A supplement that may help you ease tension while you are working through, and resolving, the stress in your life is kava-kava (kava for short), available in health food stores and pharmacies without a doctor's prescription. Kava is a relatively new herb to the United States but not in Germany, where it has been available for decades. In 1990, the German Commission approved kava for treating anxiety, stress, and restlessness.

Significantly, kava's benefits have been verified by extensive research. One of the most recent studies was conducted in the United States. Researchers at Virginia Commonwealth University measured the effects of kava on the everyday hassles of life and found that the supplement had remarkable stress-relieving benefits.

A member of the pepper family, kava has been around for thousands of years in the South Pacific as part of a water-based drink used in religious and social rites. The herb's therapeutic effects are due to a variety of biological compounds, collectively known as kavalactones. Most of these produce physical and mental relaxation but without harmful side effects.

Kava is available in several forms: capsules, liquids, bulk, teas, standardized extracts, single herb, and multiherb. As for supplementation, abide by the manufacturer's recommended dosage. Unless under medical supervision, do not supplement with kava for longer than three months at a time. Neither should you take kava while on prescription mood medications or antihistamines—due to possibly dangerous interactions.

KOMBUCHA TEA

A beverage drunk in Asia and Russia, kombucha tea is made by fermenting special yeasts and bacteria in sweetened black or green tea. This mixture yields a jellylike blob called a Manchurian "mushroom" that floats on top of the tea. The mushroom (which is not really a mushroom) gives birth to a second blob, which can be used to produce more tea.

Kombucha tea contains various nutrients believed to help fight aging, AIDS, cancer, multiple sclerosis, and hair loss. But most of the evidence supporting kombucha tea's effectiveness is anecdotal, not scientific.

Commercial kombucha tea-making kits are available, and many herbal companies sell the tea in bottled form.

A serious problem with kombucha tea, however, is that it can become easily contaminated by poisonous microorganisms because of the way it is cultured. Also, the tea is high in plant acids, which are harmful to your health when consumed in large quantities. Thus, if you want to try the tea, drink small amounts only.

In addition, certain people should avoid kombucha tea altogether: children, the elderly, pregnant or lactating women, anyone who is ill or allergic to antibiotics, and anyone with an impaired liver or compromised immune system.

LICORICE (GLYCYRRHIZA GLABRA)

You probably think of licorice as a black, chewy candy, but it is also an herb that appears to inhibit the conversion of testosterone to DHT. Licorice is derived from the roots and underground stem of a European plant and available in capsules, powders, lozenges, and extracts.

The active compound in licorice responsible for its therapeutic benefits is glycyrrhizin, which gives the herb its sweetness. Also, licorice contains an antioxidant that may help prevent hardening of the arteries, technically known as atherosclerosis.

Supplementing with high or long-term doses of licorice extracts containing glycyrrhizin is dangerous since it may aggravate heart, liver, or kidney problems. A modified form of licorice called DGL is considered safer for use.

PUMPKIN (*CUCURBITA PEPONIS SEMEN*) SEED OIL

A common salad oil produced in Eastern bloc countries, pumpkin seed oil has garnered a lot of attention lately for its many beneficial properties. It contains disease-fighting antioxidants such as vitamin E and selenium, as well as anti-inflammatory agents, and is high in essential fats that enhance the health of hair, skin, and nails.

The German Commission E Monographs state that pumpkin seeds and other preparations (such as the oil) can be used to treat bladder conditions and to relieve symptoms of benign prostatic hypertrophy (BPH) in men.

Some alternative medicine practitioners theorize that pumpkin seed oil may influence the activity of testosterone by inhibiting the formation of the enzyme, 5 alpha-reductase. If so, it could be helpful in treating androgenetic alopecia. To date, though, no experiments investigating the supplement's potential antiandrogen nature have been conducted. However, researchers have just begun to study pumpkin oil, so we may learn more about it in the future.

PYGEUM (*PYGEUM AFRICANUM*)

Derived from the bark of an African evergreen tree, *Pygeum africanum* is used widely in Europe to treat benign prostatic hypertrophy (BPH), an enlargement of the prostate gland. Its benefit in treating BPH has been verified by scientific research spanning three decades.

Pygeum africanum works by disabling the enzyme 5 alpha-reductase, which converts testosterone into DHT. The herb also exerts an anti-inflammatory effect.

Men seeking natural cures for baldness are turning to *Pygeum africanum*—often with satisfying results. However, the herb has not been specifically tested as an antibaldness remedy. No one yet knows whether it can help women with thinning hair.

SAW PALMETTO (*SERONOA REPENS*)

Taking center stage as a potential natural remedy for baldness is saw palmetto. This herb is extracted from the berries of the fan palm, native to the eastern seaboard of the United States. In Germany, it is one of several plants approved to help men with benign prostatic hypertrophy (BPH). Extensive research confirms that saw palmetto helps increase urinary flow, cuts the frequency of urination, and makes it easier to pass urine. Several herbal medicines containing saw palmetto are marketed in Europe.

The herb prevents DHT from locking on to cellular receptor sites in the hair follicle and in the prostate gland. It also foils the action of 5 alpha-reductase, which converts testosterone to DHT. The net effect is to block the formation of DHT and prevent it from damaging the follicles.

Saw palmetto has not been specifically tested as a hair-loss remedy. Further, this herb is generally taken by men and should probably be avoided by women until more is known about how it works.

SESAME (*SESAMUM INDICUM*)

Eating sesame seeds to treat baldness is an old Chinese remedy. However, there's no scientific evidence available to recommend sesame as a treatment for thinning hair.

Sesame seeds are a healthy food, though, because they are high in cholesterol-lowering compounds called phytosterols and contain plenty of disease-fighting antioxidants.

STINGING NETTLE (*UTICA DIOICA*)

Stinging nettle is among the quartet of herbs used in Germany to treat benign prostatic hypertrophy (BPH) in men. The other herbs are saw palmetto, *Pygeum africanum*, and pumpkin seed oil.

As is the case with all these herbs, extracts of stinging nettle have been found to block the conversion of DHT into testosterone. This herb is also rich in the mineral boron, known to support hair health.

Practitioners of herbal medicine in Germany feel that stinging nettle can help prevent thinning and balding hair in men. But there are no studies supporting this claim, and no one knows if the herb can help women with thinning hair.

However, nettle steeped in water and used as a hair rinse can boost your hair volume. Let four tablespoons of the dried herb simmer in a cup of water for about thirty minutes. Strain and cool, then pour it over your hair.

The herb has other healing applications. Throughout the world, it's used to treat allergies, asthma, and bronchitis.

Oral Herbal Dosages

If you decide to supplement with any of these herbs, how much should you take? Actually, no exact dosages have been determined for treating hair loss in women. But if you want to supplement, do not exceed the dosages recommended on the label. For further information, follow these safety guidelines:

1. Do not take any herbs if you are pregnant or lactating.
2. Educate yourself on herbal therapies and the research, if any, behind them.
3. Purchase herbal supplements from well-known, reputable companies.

4. Look for supplements that are "standardized." Use of this term means that the product has been processed to ensure a uniform level of one or more isolated active ingredients from batch to batch. To standardize a product, the manufacturer extracts key active ingredients from the whole herb, measures them, sometimes concentrates them, and then formulates them in a base with other nutrients, including the whole herb. Standardization is a good guarantee of product quality.

5. Read the labels on any herb you might purchase. Make sure you know what each ingredient is and what effect it has on the body. Don't buy the supplement until you've learned all you can about its ingredients and its potential side effects.

6. Inform your doctor that you are taking an herbal supplement, especially during an illness or before surgery or if you have a preexisting medical condition. If you don't communicate this information, you're risking the chance that your doctor may unwittingly prescribe something that will interact dangerously with the supplement.

7. Follow the manufacturer's or doctor's suggestion regarding dosage. Also, pay close attention to any warnings or precautions that appear on the supplement label.

8. Report any adverse effects to your physician.

9. As with medicines, regard any herb as potentially harmful to children and keep them safely out of sight.

Herbs for Topical Use

ALOE (ALOE VERA)

A member of the lily family, aloe is an African succulent plant. Its leaves are filled with an antibacterial and antifungal gel that appears to be useful as a topical agent for treating wounds and healing first- and second-degree burns, as well as X-ray or radiation burns. The gel also acts as an anti-inflammatory agent and contains a number of helpful chemicals that naturally stimulate the immune system.

A study on aloe vera as a treatment for psoriasis revealed that the herb activates the production of nitric oxide—a messenger-like substance that appears to signal hair to grow. In addition, aloe contains a health-protecting antioxidant enzyme called "superoxide dismutase." Some investigators have theorized that nitric oxide and superoxide dismutase, working in partnership, may stimulate hair regrowth in androgenetic alopecia.

Also, some sufferers of alopecia areata have used aloe to help relieve inflammation in the hair follicles. However, aloe vera is not a baldness cure by any means.

ONION (*ALLIUM CEPA*)

You chop it up for spaghetti sauce, slice it for hamburgers, mix it in sour cream for dip, but did you ever think of using onion as a hair tonic?

The versatile onion is loaded with sulfur, a hair-healing mineral. Some herbalists recommend rubbing half a raw onion into your scalp before washing your hair. They swear it is a very effective treatment for scalp and hair problems—and that it might even stimulate hair growth. It certainly can't hurt, so you might want to give it a try. But unfortunately, there's no proof or scientific guarantee that raw onion will enhance hair growth.

RED PEPPER (*CAPSICUM*)

Red pepper is a spicy plant used to season various foods. It's also a rich source of antioxidants and contains a natural painkiller known as capsaicin.

Applying a poultice of red pepper to the scalp is an old folk remedy for treating alopecia areata. Red pepper irritates the scalp, provoking inflammation. This reaction is believed to stimulate hair growth. The application of irritation-inducing drugs is a bona fide treatment for alopecia areata (see pages 77–79), but no experiments have ever proved red pepper's value in this regard.

Capsicum extract, diluted with water, can be used as a hair rinse to invigorate the scalp.

ROSEMARY (*ROSEMARINUS OFFICINALIS*)

Men and women down through the ages have massaged rosemary and oils into their scalps to promote healthy hair. Even today, you find rosemary as an ingredient in many hair care products. But is there any scientific evidence backing its use?

Possibly. In a recent study conducted at the Aberdeen Royal Infirmary in Scotland, forty-three people with alopecia areata received daily two-minute scalp massages with essential oils of rosemary, thyme, lavender, and cedarwood blended with jojoba and grapeseed oils. A control group of forty-three people received massages with jojoba and grapeseed oils only.

After seven months of massage treatment, nineteen people in the essential oil group regrew hair, compared to only six people in the control group. Amazingly, one man grew a full head of hair after being nearly bald!

It's not clear why the essential oil massage worked so well, or which herbs were responsible for the improvement. Rosemary, however, has a couple of proven merits. It contains two antioxidants—carnosol and carnosic acid—that actively protect cells from attack by free radicals.

Thus, rosemary is one of many herbs that helps protect your immune system, and in doing so, may help prevent hair loss. In addition, rosemary is believed to help reduce oiliness in the hair and scalp when applied as part of a rinse.

Rosemary is approved by the German Commission E as an internal treatment for stomach complaints and as an external treatment for joint and circulatory problems.

SAFFLOWER (*CARTHAMUS TINCTORIUS*)

Asian health care practitioners believe that safflower is a vasodilator, an agent that opens up blood vessels, including those in the scalp. With blood vessels dilated, more nutrients can make their way to hair follicles. Safflower oil is usually applied topically and massaged into the scalp. The massaging action helps increase the delivery of nutrients to follicles, too.

Safflower oil is also rich in linoleic acid, an essential fat that enhances the condition of your hair.

Sage (*Salvia officinalis*)

You know sage best as a flavoring used to spice up turkey and dressing at Thanksgiving. But did you also know that it's a folk medicine believed to prevent hair loss and preserve hair color?

That's right: Sage, along with its Asian relative danshen (red sage), has an age-old reputation as a hair restorer. Today, you find it as an ingredient in hair care products and nonprescription antibaldness ointments. But whether it lives up to its folkloric reputation has not yet been confirmed by medical experiments.

Sage is listed in the German Commission E Monographs as an external treatment for inflammation of the mucous membranes of the nose and throat, and as an internal medication for stomach problems and excessive perspiration.

HERBAL INGREDIENTS IN HAIR CARE PRODUCTS

Many commercial shampoos, conditioners, and other hair care products contain herbs and plant extracts. If your hair is thinning, do they do any good?

Probably—because they're mild and less irritating to the scalp. Unless your dermatologist prescribes a certain shampoo, it's best to select natural shampoos containing as few chemicals as possible. Choosing an herbal shampoo is a step in the right direction.

All shampoos contain a basic detergent, usually listed on the label as a sulfate. It cleanses the hair and gives the shampoo its lather. Beyond the detergent, there are some common herbal ingredients that can enhance your hair care program. Here is a rundown:

Balsam

This is a resinous substance extracted from herbs grown in South America. Balsam adds body, strength, and volume to hair—three desirable qualities when your hair is thinning. Balsam also reduces oily buildup on the scalp.

Chamomile

Ranked as one of the top five herbs used worldwide, chamomile grows on meadows in North America, Europe, North Africa, and parts of Asia. Chamomile is a member of the daisy family. Although usually enjoyed as a tea, chamomile has found its way into hair care products, particularly because it brings out distinctive blond highlights in hair. You can make your own rinse simply by preparing a cup or two of chamomile tea and pouring it (cooled) over your hair. Chamomile is also very soothing to the scalp.

Henna

The active ingredient in the henna plant is hennatannic acid, which coats hair fibers to help seal in the hair's natural oils. Henna is an ingredient in many natural hair care products.

Plant Oils

Used as conditioning agents, these include wheat germ, jojoba, coconut, and avocado oils. They restore your hair's natural moisture and patch up cuticles roughed up by heat, chemicals, and sun exposure. Pure jojoba oil, in particular, is an excellent remedy for soothing a dry, flaky scalp.

Shea Butter

A relatively new ingredient finding its way into hair products, shea comes from the seed of an African tree that is related to the coconut. Shea butter, or oil, is water-soluble and acts as a moisturizer. It has a reputation of making hair silkier and shinier.

Tea Tree Oil

This popular herbal is a natural antiseptic that fights bacteria and heals irritated skin. As an ingredient in herbal shampoos, it's good for normal to dry hair. Tea tree oil-based shampoos can also help prevent dandruff.

Hair Savers: What the Experts Recommend

Emily A. Kane, N.D., L.Ac.
Doctor of Naturopathic Medicine
Licensed Acupuncturist

Dr. Kane is the former editor of the *Journal of Naturopathic Medicine* as well as one of its contributors. She also writes for the *Townsend Letter for Doctors & Patients, Choices,* and *Let's Live Magazine.* Dr. Kane practices naturopathic medicine, lectures frequently (especially on breast cancer prevention and optimal nutrition), and teaches yoga. In addition, she has nine years of postgraduate training, including medical residencies.

For women experiencing hair loss, Dr. Kane generally recommends the following:

• 8,000 micrograms (8 milligrams) of biotin daily for six weeks. "Biotin is an extremely safe vitamin, even for lactating mothers, with no known side effects," she says. "Check with your health care provider for an individualized dosage."

• One cup daily of horsetail tea (*Equisetum arvense*) for its mineral content, particularly silica.

• Limited intake of refined foods in your diet.

• An exercise in which you stand on your head three to seven times weekly for twenty-five to forty breaths. "While this may sound crazy, it actually helps to bring fresh blood to the scalp," Dr. Kane explains.

Although individual results vary, you may begin to see an improvement in the condition of your hair within a month.

THIRTEEN

Special Hair-Saving Supplements

I F YOU ARE experiencing hair loss and are undergoing treatment for it, you may want to explore the use of some special supplements as supportive therapy. Here are some for you to consider:

Bee Pollen

Remember the healthy head of hair sported by President Ronald Reagan? Reportedly, the former president supplemented with bee pollen.

Bee pollen is actually a loose powder of bee saliva, plant nectar, and pollen compressed into tablets of 400 to 500 milligrams or poured into capsules. It also comes in pellets to be sprinkled on foods. Often, bee pollen is formulated with other supplements.

Bee pollen is rich in amino acids, with a protein content that averages 20 percent but ranges from 10 to 36 percent. This supplement also contains varying amounts of B-complex vitamins, biotin, inositol, calcium, silicon, and sulfur—all of great importance to hair.

If you supplement, follow the manufacturer's recommended dosage. Bee pollen is a natural food, but it does contain pollen.

That means you could have an allergic reaction if you're prone to allergies.

Brewer's Yeast

Brewer's yeast, or nutritional yeast, is a rich source of B vitamins, especially vitamin B_{12}, and can be used as a B-complex supplement. Because our highly refined diets are so devoid of these nutrients, brewer's yeast is a highly nutritious way to add them back in.

Brewer's yeast is also a treasure trove of amino acids, minerals, and other vitamins. Its protein quality, which refers to how well protein is absorbed and used by the body, is equivalent to that of steak or eggs.

Brewer's yeast is an excellent source of RNA, a nucleic acid that protects the body against degenerative diseases, including dry and wrinkling skin. This supplement can also protect against the adverse side effects of hormones.

Available in powder or flakes, brewer's yeast can be added to other foods. Admittedly, its flavor takes some getting used to, but you'll find that it tastes best in tomato juice, soups, and cereals. It also comes in tablets. The recommended supplemental allowance of brewer's yeast is one or two tablespoons daily, or follow the manufacturer's recommended dose.

Co-Enzyme Q_{10}

Technically known as ubiquinone, coenzyme Q_{10} (abbreviated as CoQ_{10}) is found naturally within cells, where it is involved in the conversion of food to energy. Supplementally, it is a nutrient that appears to have many health-giving properties. For example, it helps improve cardiac function, strengthens the immune system, and may enhance the quality of overall health.

As for hair health, coenzyme Q_{10} helps promote blood circulation, including circulation to the scalp. People who supplement with it feel that it makes their hair thicker and more vibrant.

There are no studies that prove this benefit, however. Nonetheless, CoQ$_{10}$ is a good all-around supplement that supports health. For best results, supplement with 20 to 30 milligrams daily.

Desiccated Liver

One of the best dietary moves you can make to nourish your body with hair-healthy nutrients is to eat liver once or twice a week. But who can choke it down? Among most people, liver is not high on the list of favorite foods. Plus, it's overloaded with cholesterol and saturated fat.

An alternative to eating liver is to take desiccated liver supplements, available in tablets or powder. Desiccated liver is a concentrated source of liver that has been processed to remove all the fat and cholesterol. With four times the nutritional value in the same amount of cooked whole liver, this supplemental food is rich in protein; vitamins A, B, and C; and the minerals calcium, phosphorus, and heme iron. Heme iron is a type of iron derived from animal proteins that is well absorbed by the body. In fact, the absorption rate of heme iron is as high as 35 percent, compared to 5 percent for non-heme iron (obtained from plant sources). Depending on the supplement, desiccated liver contains about 2 milligrams of iron (the recommended daily intake is 15 milligrams), so you don't have to worry about ingesting too much iron.

Follow the supplement manufacturer's dosage recommendation. You can enrich soups, stews, and other foods by adding desiccated liver powder to the recipe.

Dimethylglycine (DMG)

Dimethylglycine (DMG) is derived from glycine, an amino acid that is highly concentrated in the skin and connective tissues. Supplementing with DMG has a number of health-boosting benefits. It enhances your immune system, reduces levels of harmful blood fats in the body, and helps normalize blood pressure and blood sugar. Where hair is concerned, DMG may help improve scalp circulation to keep your hair well supplied with oxygen and nutrients. The recommended dosage is 100 milligrams daily.

Essential Fatty Acid Supplements (EFAs)

Essential fatty acids (EFAs) are vitaminlike substances that have a protective effect on the body. The reason they are called "essential" is because your body cannot manufacture them; you must obtain them from the foods you eat. They have very specific roles to play in maintaining health.

EFAs, for example, protect the integrity of cell walls, making them flexible enough so that important materials such as nutrients and hormones can be exchanged from inside and outside the cell. Without adequate EFAs, cell walls become too rigid, and materials cannot easily pass in and out.

EFAs also help mobilize cholesterol and other harmful fats from the body. If EFAs are unavailable, cholesterol molecules latch on to saturated fat molecules and can end up as plaque on the inner wall of the arteries.

EFAs are also needed to produce prostaglandins. These are hormonelike substances that regulate nearly every system in your body, including your cardiovascular, immune, endocrine, central nervous, digestive, and reproductive systems. When EFAs are in ample supply, your entire body functions much better. In addition, immunity to disease and infection is greatly increased.

Signs of an EFA deficiency are hair loss; dry, flaky skin; and stiff, painful joints. These symptoms may indicate that your heart, brain, liver, and internal organs are EFA-deficient as well.

You can obtain EFAs by supplementing with natural essential fats, namely black currant, Evening Primrose, and borage oils. These are loaded with gamma-linolenic acid, a nutrient that has a hand in promoting healthy skin, hair, and nails. In animal studies, gamma-linolenic acid and other unsaturated fats have been found to block the activity of 5 alpha-reductase, the enzyme that converts testosterone into follicle-damaging DHT.

If your hair is thinning, many alternative health care practitioners recommend taking 500 milligrams of one of these supplements each day. You should notice an improvement in hair health in about six to eight weeks.

Always take EFAs in supplemental form. Cooking these fats destroys the fatty acids and can spawn dangerous free radicals in the process.

An animal fat high in the EFA linolenic acid is emu oil, sold as a topical hair restorer. In mice studies, emu oil applied to the skin stimulated hair follicle development and growth. Some people who have used emu oil report good results, though scientific tests using humans are needed to confirm its benefits.

Methylsulfonylmethane (MSM)

Methylsulfonylmethane (MSM) is a form of organic sulfur found in vegetables, meat, poultry, eggs, and dairy foods. Its job in the body is to make enzymes, antibodies, and antioxidants. It is also involved in producing the structural tissue found in hair, nails, and skin. Along with other sulfur compounds, MSM is used by the body to make protein.

Some MSM in food is destroyed by processing, which is why many alternative health care practitioners recommend supplementation. MSM has been used successfully to treat allergies; heal wounds; and relieve the pain and stiffness of arthritis. People who take MSM say it makes their hair stronger, thicker, and shinier.

If you supplement with MSM, the recommended dosage is two 1,000-milligram tablets daily with food. MSM also comes as a skin lotion to soothe achy joints.

Royal Jelly

Royal jelly is a white, milky substance produced by worker bees and fed to the bee destined to become the queen. In fact, the royal jelly "dinner" is what turns an ordinary bee into a queen bee—an insect that's larger, more fertile, and longer-lived.

Sold in capsules, royal jelly is a rich source of pantothenic acid, a B-complex vitamin involved in releasing energy from foods and in protecting the body against cellular damage. Royal jelly is also loaded with amino acids; vitamins A, C, D, and E; hair-healthy minerals such as calcium, iron, sulfur, and silica; and the nucleic acid RNA. In addition, royal jelly contains a substance called "globulinic acid," which builds resistance to bacteria and viruses and stimulates the immune system.

Taking royal jelly reportedly improves the health of hair and makes it glossier. One reason is that it abounds in the amino acid cystine, an important constituent of hair. Because it acts as an emollient and a moisturizer, royal jelly is also an ingredient in many topical skin care products.

When supplementing with royal jelly, follow the manufacturer's dosage recommendations. A note of caution: In susceptible individuals, royal jelly may provoke an allergic reaction.

Viviscal—A Miracle Marine Supplement with Antibaldness Powers

Viviscal is a natural food supplement formulated with the mineral silica, credited with the ability to build healthy hair. Launched in Finland in 1992, Viviscal also contains a fish oil extract. To its credit, the product is backed by several scientific studies conducted in Europe and Latin America. One of these studies tested Viviscal against a product containing fish oil extract only. Lasting six months, the study involved twenty men who took two tablets of Viviscal daily and twenty who received two tablets of the fish oil extract daily.

The results were intriguing: After six months, the Viviscal-treated group grew 38 percent more hair, compared to just 2 percent in the other group. The researchers noted that "Viviscal appears to be the first highly active treatment for androgenetic alopecia in young males."

It's not clear why the product worked so well, but the common denominator may have been silica. The control supplement, which produced no results, was free of silica. In addition, researchers believe that the mixture of ingredients in the supplement may help reactivate the resting hair follicle to get hair growing again.

Available information on the product states that it's formulated for both men and women. It may be worth a try, and you can order it from: www.viviscal.com. The supplement costs between $38 and $78 a month.

Purchasing Quality Supplements

Nutritional supplements are not regulated or approved by the FDA as prescription drugs are, so it's hard to know whether or not you're buying a quality product. A good rule of thumb is to try to find brands from well-known manufacturers such as pharmaceutical companies. Finally, if you choose to supplement, follow the manufacturer's dosage recommendation and always get your doctor's blessing before supplementing.

PART 5

Hair

to

Stay

FOURTEEN

Surgical Help for Troubled Tresses

YOU CAN TREAT baldness and thinning hair permanently—
with hair restoration surgery. It's one of the most
commonly performed cosmetic procedures in the world,
especially in men. Only 5 to 10 percent of all hair restoration
surgery is done in women.

That's not to say this surgery does not work well for women. It
does. However, there are limitations. Hair restoration surgery
takes hair you already have and moves it to areas of less hair. This
gives the illusion of more hair, but you still have the same amount
of hair. It has just been redistributed. Most men can live with this,
but a lot of women can't. They want more hair. This is why it is
important to learn as much as you can about this form of cosmetic surgery—what it can and can't do for you.

There are various types of hair restoration surgery, including
hair transplantation, scalp reductions, flaps, and expanders.

Hair Transplantation

Among the most exciting advances in the treatment of hair loss
today are found in the area of hair transplants. Today, sophisti-
cated techniques in the hands of skilled cosmetic surgeons are
producing stunning results for women who take this route.

In hair transplantation, areas of scalp with healthy hair follicles (*donor sites*) are surgically transplanted onto bald patches (*recipient sites*). This procedure is also called *hair grafting*. It was developed in the 1930s by a Japanese dermatologist and first described in American medical literature in 1959.

Transplanted hair is taken from the back and sides of the scalp. The hair follicles located there are not affected by the hormones that trigger androgenetic alopecia. Therefore, hair is less likely to fall out and should continue to grow, even after being relocated to another part of the scalp.

Are You a Good Candidate for a Hair Transplant?

Until about ten years ago, many surgeons considered women with thinning hair unsuitable candidates for hair transplantation surgery. Not anymore. Thanks to developments and refinements in surgical techniques, many women can benefit from hair transplantation. Here's a look at the major factors that determine the results you'll achieve from a hair transplant.

DEGREE OF HAIR THINNING

A hair transplant is a permanent solution to baldness, but it's possible only if you have enough hair to spare from the back or sides of your scalp. Very diffuse thinning all over your scalp may make a hair transplant inadvisable. However, a technique called the *slit graft* (see page 192) can produce natural-looking results even in cases of diffuse thinning.

TYPE OF ALOPECIA

Hair transplants are performed mostly on patients with androgenetic alopecia or with permanent baldness caused by burns or infection, but usually not on patients with alopecia areata. With alopecia areata, there's always the chance that your hair will grow back on its own. Furthermore, patients with alopecia totalis or alopecia universalis do not have enough donor hair to warrant the procedure.

HAIR QUALITY

The quality of your existing hair is important. Hair that's broken or diseased does not produce pleasing transplant results. The surgeon can judge the quality of your hair by examining it under a microscope.

CURL

Is your hair naturally curly? Then you're in luck. Curly hair covers the scalp better than straight hair, for two reasons. First, it twists and turns as soon as it emerges from the follicle, and thus spreads out over the graft to give better scalp coverage. Second, curly hair naturally creates the illusion of more hair. Wavy hair gives good results, too. Straight hair does not cover as well.

TEXTURE

On average, hair is coarse, fine, or somewhere in between. Transplanted coarse hair covers well but is less manageable. Sometimes it looks less natural because it contrasts too much with the skin. On the other hand, fine hair does not cover the scalp as well, though it gives a natural look because of its low contrast with the skin.

HAIR AND SKIN COLOR

The closer your hair color is to your skin color, the better your scalp coverage will look. Gray, blond, red, and light brown hair tend to look more natural because there is usually less contrast to the skin. Also, if you have black hair and black skin, you'll get a very natural appearance. On the other hand, black hair and dark brown hair can overly contrast with a lighter complexion and thus produce less pleasing results. Darker hair colors often require more transplant sessions to soften the contrast.

According to Edmond Griffin, M.D., writing in the 1995 issue of *Dermatologic Clinics*: "The best patients for hair replacement are those with Celtic or Irish backgrounds (blond, light brown, and red hair) and graying patients. These patients show the lowest skin-to-hair contrast and regardless of their other hair characteristics of wave, caliber and density, show the least grafting difficulties."

AGE

Age is a critical factor. Most surgeons don't like to perform transplant surgery in men or women under the age of thirty because it's hard to predict the future course of their balding. If you're younger than age thirty, you should consider other alternatives, such as prescription medications or a hair system, before undergoing any type of surgery.

By the time you're in your late thirties or forties, however, it's easier to tell how extensive your hair loss will be. The ideal candidate for a hair transplant is in her forties or older. Your surgeon should design your transplant to look not only natural now but also when you're well into your fifties, sixties, and beyond.

GENERAL HEALTH

Your medical history and health habits determine whether you're a good candidate for a hair transplant. Generally, the healthier you are, the better the transplant will go. By contrast, certain habits can adversely affect hair growth following a transplant. Smoking marijuana, for example, has been found to retard hair growth in transplanted hair.

Realistic Expectations

Balding takes more of an emotional and psychological toll on women than it does on men. Thus, we can be hard to please and more easily disappointed if a hair transplant doesn't meet our expectations.

If you are considering hair restoration surgery, approach it realistically. Foremost, keep in mind that this type of surgery can't restore your hair to the dense, lush locks of your youth.

"The goal of all hair restoration surgery is to produce a fullness that will look natural as the individual ages," cautioned Robert M. Bernstein, M.D., a pioneer in the field, in the January 1996 issue of *Dermatologic Surgery*. "An attempt to match or exceed one's original density, even if only at the frontal hairline, will not only be cosmetically unacceptable in the long term, but will tax the donor bank and limit the ability to cover additional areas as the balding progresses."

Your surgeon should clearly explain to you the limitations of a hair transplant, including the fact that you could experience further thinning in the future. The progression of balding is very unpredictable. If you can't accept the limitations of the procedure, you may want to reconsider.

AN OVERVIEW OF THE HAIR TRANSPLANT PROCEDURE

Once your surgeon has determined you're an appropriate candidate for a hair transplant, you'll be scheduled for a presurgery visit about two weeks prior to your operation. During this visit, you'll have routine blood tests (including the HIV and hepatitis B screens), go over any allergies and medical conditions with your surgeon, review the surgical plan, get answers to any last-minute questions, and sign consents.

In addition, your surgeon will probably ask you about any medications you're taking. Aspirin, alcohol, warfarin (Coumadin), vitamin E, and vitamin E–containing products may increase bleeding during surgery. Thus, it's wise to avoid these products for a few weeks prior to your operation.

You should also discuss your hair-styling preferences with your surgeon, since hair transplants can often be designed to accommodate your hairstyle. The presurgery visit usually takes about two hours.

Your own hair is used for the transplant. This was not always the case. In the 1970s, synthetic hairlike fibers were inserted into bald areas of the scalp. But this type of procedure was banned by the FDA in 1984 because it caused infection, permanent scarring, and other complications.

The operation is performed by the surgeon, who is aided by a team of surgical assistants. You're sedated and given local anesthesia to numb your scalp. Some surgeons use music to help relax their patients. The donor and recipient areas of the scalp will be cleansed with special antiseptics.

The operation takes several hours. Generally, the hairline and top of your scalp receive transplanted hair, also referred to as *grafts*. These vary in size and shape. Hair is transplanted onto the crown later, unless that is the only balding area on your head. It takes approximately five hundred or more grafts to cover a three-inch-square area of scalp.

After the operation, your head remains bandaged (usually in a turbanlike dressing) for at least a day, and you may have to take painkillers or antibiotics. You'll be given a detailed set of postoperative instructions on diet, sleep posture (there is less tendency to bleed if you keep your head elevated), activity, shampooing, and hair grooming. You should follow these instructions to the letter to avoid complications.

Further operations are usually required to achieve a natural look. Some surgeons, however, will do an entire procedure in one day. This is called a *megasession*, and it lasts roughly eight hours.

The cost of a hair implant varies widely, but a typical session runs somewhere between $3,500 and $5,000. So if you have two sessions, which is the average, you could spend roughly $10,000. If your hair loss is extensive, expect to pay around $20,000.

Because they are considered cosmetic surgery, hair transplantation and other hair restoration surgeries are not normally covered by health insurance. However, if your hair loss is the result of a disease, accident, burn, or physical trauma, surgery may be reimbursable. Check with your insurance agent or health care provider.

Hair Grafts

There are several types of hair grafts, some superior to others. Before considering a hair implant, educate yourself about the various types of procedures and ask your plastic surgeon which one is best for your personal situation—and why.

ROUND OR SQUARE GRAFTS

The very first type of hair grafting developed was the punch graft technique. Three- to five-millimeter circular or square plugs, consisting of ten to twenty hairs each, are removed from the hair-bearing site and planted, one by one, into smaller cylindrical or square holes in the balding region of the scalp. The surgeon uses a special tubelike steel instrument to punch out the round graft at the donor site so that it can be transplanted at the recipient site.

This procedure is an older, outdated transplant method that fails to duplicate the appearance of a natural, hair-bearing scalp. The problem with these grafts is that they make your scalp look like doll hair—pluggy sprigs of hair coming out of the scalp—an unnatural appearance. Yet this procedure has been used successfully to correct the hairlines of African-American women who have lost hair due to traction alopecia.

Fortunately, these larger grafts have evolved into smaller and smaller grafts, which give a more natural-looking appearance and better long-term results.

MINIGRAFTS

More recently, surgeons have started using smaller versions of grafts called *minigrafts* and *micrografts*. With minigrafts, the surgeon uses a scalpel to remove thin strips of hair-bearing scalp from the back and sides of the head and cuts them into small rectangles or circles of three to eight follicles each. These plugs are then inserted into shallow incisions on the scalp. In a three-hour operation, up to a thousand graphs can be placed in these incisions.

From minigrafts evolved micrografts, which consist of one to three hairs inserted into needle holes. Micrografts have a number of advantages over the larger punch grafts. For example:

- Less clumpiness on the scalp
- Faster healing and better hair growth
- Minimal scarring
- Versatility (Micrografts can be used in a variety of alopecias.)

Both minigrafts and micrografts are used to soften the front hairline and are meant to mask the "doll's hair" appearance of larger grafts. The fewer hairs per graft, the easier it is to achieve a more natural look. Even so, some surgeons feel that minigrafts do not match the way hair grows in nature.

In studies of mini- and micrografting, the procedure has been found to be safe, without serious complications. Patients who have undergone these procedures are usually very satisfied with the results. In addition, women with gray or blond hair, as well as African Americans, are good candidates for minigrafts.

LINEAR OR LINE GRAFTS

In this procedure, the surgeon removes a three- to four-millimeter strip, or line, of donor hair from the back or sides of the scalp. A trench is cut into the bald area, and the entire donor strip, or a major portion of it, is grafted onto the bald areas. Several sessions are usually required. The result of this type of procedure is usually not cosmetically pleasing.

SLIT GRAFTS

There is a relatively new advance in linear grafting called the *slit graft*, which consists of grafts of three to four hairs. Slits look more natural than holes created by a punch and work well in women who have diffuse thinning regions of hair. Slit grafts, as well as minigrafts, are scattered uniformly throughout the balding areas to create the optical illusion of more hair.

A line of grafts is removed from the donor site, which is then stitched or stapled closed. Each graft is inserted into a slit, rather than into a round hole, made by a scalpel or laser. Slit grafts allow hair to grow in its natural direction. In addition, it creates a denser, more natural-looking appearance because the recipient site exactly matches the size of the donor graft—a benefit not achieved with conventional linear grafts. Slit grafts are a good way to fill in a thinning hairline. They are also used in conjunction with punch graphs and to fill in the spaces created in between previously placed punch grafts.

In general, three to five operations are necessary, spaced at least three months apart to allow for adequate healing.

FOLLICULAR UNIT TRANSPLANTATION

The newest and most advanced method of grafting is a procedure called *follicular unit transplantation*. It's based on the fact that your hair grows in natural clusters of one to four terminal (normal) hairs each. These clusters are termed *follicular units*. Each unit also contains one or two vellus hairs, sebaceous glands, fat tissue, and some collagen.

In follicular unit transplantation, the surgeon harvests hair in these naturally occurring units and grafts them to balding sections of the scalp. The goal is to place and distribute these units in such a way that cosmetically pleasing results are achieved.

Developed by hair transplant pioneers Robert M. Bernstein, M.D., and William R. Rassman, M.D., the procedure offers numerous advantages over other types of hair transplants:

• Fuller-looking hair
• Faster healing
• Better hair growth
• No pluggy, doll hair–like appearance
• Natural-looking results

If you elect to have a follicular unit transplant, here's generally what to expect while undergoing the procedure:

First, you'll probably receive a sedative to relax you and a local anesthetic to numb your scalp. Next, the surgeon will select a donor strip of scalp with healthy hair follicles and remove it using a scalpel. As with other grafting procedures, the donor strip is usually taken from the back or sides of the head. The strip is temporarily preserved in a special saline solution. The surgeon stitches up the donor area to close the wound, which should heal in about a week or two. You'll have a slight scar, but it will be barely visible.

Medical technicians dissect the donor strip to remove any extra fat tissue and then cut it into hundreds of follicular units of one to four hairs each. To prepare the recipient site, the surgeon creates a tiny incision using a specialized needle. Unlike other hair transplant procedures, no slits or holes are required to accept the donor strip. The recipient sites created in follicular unit transplantation are smaller than holes or slits produced by any other method of hair transplantation.

The follicular units are then placed on the recipient site in a direction that matches the natural growth of your hair. Placement is usually done manually with forceps, or performed with a newer surgical instrument called the Rapid Fire Hair Implanter Carousel, which is a disposable, hand-held device that houses the individual follicular grafts. It has a sharp end that pierces the scalp and an insertion device that moves the implants into the recipient site. The entire procedure typically lasts six to seven hours.

On average, it takes three to four months for transplanted hair to start growing. In some cases, it can take up to a year or longer. Sometimes, additional follicular transplantations are warranted, usually to further refine the hairline, add some density, or to transplant an entirely new area. If you and your surgeon determine that further sessions are needed, it's best to wait eight to twelve months between procedures, so that your transplanted hair has had time to grow.

Dilators

Before implanting the hair for a transplant procedure, some surgeons may insert a tiny, strawlike pin called a *dilator* into the slits or holes to widen them. The surgeon removes the dilator, then implants the hair in the widened hole or slit.

Dilators are not really necessary, some surgeons feel, because hair can be placed in the holes without them. Plus, they have several disadvantages. Dilators may cause the implanted hair to grow in the wrong direction, and they can cause tissue damage at the recipient site. What's more, the dilator-widened holes have to be spaced more widely apart, resulting in poor coverage. Critics argue that the routine use of dilators may be a sign that the surgeon is less skilled at performing hair implants.

Other surgeons beg to differ, arguing that the dilators, specifically a newer type that is tear-shaped, provide easier placement of grafts and fewer surgical complications.

Laser Hair Transplantation

With most hair implants, holes or slits are made in the recipient site with a surgical scalpel or other special instrument. Increasingly though, some surgeons are using highly focused laser beams to create the slits into which the grafts are inserted.

The use of laser technology for hair transplants is very new, employed for the first time in 1992. There are different types of lasers in use. One of the chief types is the pulsating laser, in which the light beam is rapidly pulsed up to hundreds of times a second. These lasers create holes by vaporizing scalp tissue, thus minimizing injury to surrounding tissue. Small amounts of bald tissue can also be removed, and this reduces the total area of baldness on the scalp. Lasers are not normally used to harvest the donor hairs.

Advocates of lasers in hair transplants say that their use reduces bleeding, prevents a lumpy look on the scalp, cuts the length of the operation, and eases patient discomfort.

However, some surgeons are not totally sold on the benefits of lasers. The downside of laser use includes more postoperative crusting on the scale, longer time to produce the slits, and delayed hair growth. With regard to the latter, at least one study has found that hair growth from laser-created sites was not as great as that from sites created with conventional surgical methods. In addition, the use of laser beams can destroy collagen and other connective tissue under the skin. This may cause grafts to fall out of their holes more easily.

If considering hair implant surgery, be sure to thoroughly discuss the pros and cons of laser technology with your surgeon.

Postfacelift Grafting

If you've had several facelifts and have lost a lot of hair at the hairline above your ears as a result, hair transplantation can correct this. Typically, surgeons use a combination of slit grafts, round grafts, and micrografts to fill in the hairline. Two or three sessions, spaced a minimum of four months apart, are usually required.

Complications of Hair Grafts

Hair grafts, like any surgical procedure, are not without risks and complications. It's critical to understand what they are before you decide to go through with surgery. In addition, be sure to discuss the risks with your surgeon. What follows is a description of potential complications.

Poor Hair Growth. Most of your implanted hair will grow, but it may take some time, depending on your rate of healing and individual factors that are not well understood.

Infection. Although extremely rare, infection may occur in the follicles—a condition called *folliculitis*. It can be easily treated with antibiotics and does not usually affect hair growth.

Fibrosis. Fibrosis is a buildup of collagen in response to tissue damage. It can set in around the donor site after hair follicles have been removed, destroying the hair adjacent to the site. This reduces the amount of potential donor hair that can be harvested for subsequent hair implants.

Each graft placed in the recipient site can also induce fibrosis, cutting off normal blood flow. Without an adequate blood supply, hair does not grow as well.

Pain. Following surgery, your scalp may hurt. The pain can last for a day or two, but can be managed with over-the-counter pain pills such as acetaminophen.

Loss of Sensation. Incisions made on the scalp may cut nerves, resulting in the loss of sensation. This can continue for several months before feeling returns.

Scarring. Significant scarring in the donor or recipient site can occur, particularly if the operation was poorly executed.

Cobblestoning. This side effect describes dents or bumps in the recipient sites where the implants are placed. They subside over time and rarely occur with follicular unit transplantation.

Cyst Formation. If you have naturally oily skin, small cysts resembling large pimples may develop in your scalp. Most likely, they are caused by tiny pieces of tissue trapped under the skin, or ingrown hairs. Cysts clear up on their own in about three or four months. Mini- and micrografting sometimes produce cysts.

Swelling. In a small percentage of patients, swelling occurs under the eyes and around the forehead. You may even have a black eye. Swelling usually lasts only three or four days, then dissipates on its own.

Temporary Hair Loss. Bodily stress such as surgery can trigger telogen effluvium, a condition in which hair goes into its resting phase and begins to shed. Don't be surprised if you experience telogen effluvium in the recipient site as a result of surgery. This loss is temporary; your hair will grow back within a few months.

In addition, there is evidence that topical minoxidil applied twice a day beginning within forty-eight hours after hair transplantation surgery minimizes shedding and stimulates faster hair growth.

What's more, a rather new treatment called GraftCyte, developed by ProCyte, appears to prevent transplanted hairs from going into a resting phase and speeds up the growth of newly grafted hair.

GraftCyte contains a copper tripeptide, a combination of copper and the amino acid lysine, that helps promote cell division in the hair matrix. GraftCyte has been approved by the FDA as a medical device for preventing hair from going into its resting stage.

With this treatment, dressings soaked in medication are placed on the transplanted area immediately after treatment and for the next several days, usually for a total of sixteen applications. The dressings are replaced every few hours and provide a moist, healing environment for the wounds—one that appears to prevent telogen effluvium.

Some surgeons use topical antibiotics as a post-transplant dressing—and even petroleum or KY jelly, both of which do a good job of keeping the new grafts moist.

Other Forms of Surgical Hair Restoration

In addition to hair transplantation, a number of other hair restoration surgeries are performed. These procedures are considered more drastic and risky.

SCALP REDUCTION

If you don't have enough donor hair to cover the bald area, your surgeon may recommend a *scalp reduction*. First introduced in 1977, this operation involves surgically removing a strip of hairless scalp to reduce the total area of baldness. Then, the remainder is pulled together and sutured closed. This reduces the bald area. Several operations may be necessary. The cost is usually $1,500 to $2,000 per procedure.

Scalp reduction surgery has been performed in conjunction with hair transplantation.

In some cases, there can be numerous complications associated with this procedure, including infection, hemorrhaging, and a long, ugly scar at the sight of the reduction. A potential side effect of scalp reduction is *stretch back*, in which the parts of the scalp that were initially pulled together and stitched lose their elasticity and stretch out. This leaves a furrowed, unsightly scar on the scalp.

Some surgeons used a technique called *minireduction*. A series of holes is punched in the recipient site and bald portions are removed. Not all the holes receive hair grafts but instead are stitched shut. This reduces the total area of baldness.

Many in the hair restoration field consider scalp reduction to be outdated and barbaric. In addition, advances in hair transplantation procedures have made them largely unnecessary.

FLAP

Flap surgery moves a flap of hair, with its tissue, hair strands, and hair follicles, to a bald area. The flap is cut on three sides, so as not to detach it from its blood supply or completely sever it from the scalp. Typically, a flap is one inch wide and three to seven inches long and can do the work of 350 punch grafts.

This procedure, however, has potential side effects:

- Tissue necrosis, in which all or part of the flap tissue dies, leaving an unsightly scar
- Infection
- An unnatural hairline
- A detectable scar along the hairline
- Hair that grows in an unnatural direction
- Loose skin in the forehead, giving a Frankenstein-like appearance

There is another type of flap surgery known as the free-form flap, in which the section of scalp is cut on four sides and placed on the balding area in the natural direction of hair growth. However, the risk of complications is just as great as with the conventional flap.

The average cost of flap surgery is $9,000 to $10,000.

SOFT TISSUE EXPANSION

In this procedure, the scalp is cut and silicone balloons are inserted under the hair-bearing area of the scalp. After the incision heals, the balloons are slowly inflated with salt water over a period of two to four months. This expands the hair-bearing skin.

Next, the bags are removed, and the bald area of the scalp is cut out. Flaps are created from the expanded hair-bearing skin.

This is a radical procedure only recommended for patients who have lost a lot of hair due to burns or traumatic scars. A potential side effect is unsightly bulges on the scalp that can last several months.

On average, this procedure costs $1,500 to 4,000.

Touch Ups

With most hair restoration surgeries, you will probably need a surgical touch-up to make your hair look even more natural. Touch-ups usually involve filling in the hairline with a combination of minigrafts, micrografts, or slit graphs. Ask your surgeon about what sort of touch-up surgery you will require.

How to Find a Qualified Surgeon

Finally, the results of your hair restoration surgery will depend largely on the skill of the surgeon you select. He or she should be uniquely qualified to perform this surgery and experienced in the field of hair restoration. What's more, a surgeon should be an artist of sorts, someone who knows how to design and plan hair restoration according to *your* unique facial aesthetics.

"Hair reconstruction is complex and requires surgical proficiency, sound medical judgment, and a creative and artistic aptitude," according to surgeons D. Bluford Stough, Barbara J. Schell, and Randall P. Weyrich, writing in the 1997 issue of *Annals of Plastic Surgery*.

Here are some important guidelines for finding a surgeon with this blend of medical expertise and artistry.

- Research and verify the surgeon's credentials. Your surgeon should be board-certified by the American Board of Hair Restoration Surgery. You can locate qualified surgeons by contacting various organizations, including the American Academy of Cosmetic Surgery (AACS), the International Society for Hair Restoration Surgeons (ISHRS), the American Hair

Loss Council (AHLC), the American Society of Plastic and Reconstructive Surgeons (ASPRS), and the American Board of Hair Restoration Surgery (ABHRS) (for contact information and website addresses, see Appendix B on page 221). Other good sources of information include your city, county, and state medical societies; your personal physician; your hair stylist; and the Better Business Bureau.

- Find out how many transplant procedures a surgeon has performed—*particularly in women.*
- Ask to see before and after photographs of patients, or better yet, talk to former patients. A surgeon should have an artistic ability for creating hairlines and filling in areas of thinning.
- Find out how many grafts you will need—and what the costs will be.
- Ask to see complication rates—the percentage of patients who have experienced complications and side effects following surgery.

Be aware, too, that there are unethical practitioners and opportunists working in the hair restoration field. Any clinic that promises a quick or easy procedure, or says you can get a full head of hair in one session, is probably out to get your money rather than improve your appearance. Don't fall prey to these gimmicks, or you'll find yourself sorely disappointed.

Hair restoration surgery is a rapidly evolving field. Improvements in technique and technology are allowing surgeons to produce better and smaller grafts, give patients a more natural appearance, and reduce surgical complications. Your challenge is to thoroughly investigate your options—and to do so rationally—before jumping into a surgery that some of the most qualified plastic surgeons still consider a calculated risk.

FIFTEEN

Nonsurgical
Hair Restoration

W ANT TO AVOID the discomfort of surgery, side effects, and the possible drain on your pocketbook? Then consider a "hair system." As defined by the American Hair Loss Council, a hair system is "any external hair-bearing device added to existing hair or scalp to give one the appearance of a fuller head of hair."

There are numerous types of hair systems available, all with the potential to greatly enhance your appearance and make you feel better about yourself.

Hair Weaving

Hair weaving is a nonsurgical option to treat thinning hair. This process involves braiding human or synthetic hair into existing hair. Several hairs are usually woven to one of your natural hairs. Your hair looks fuller and thicker as a result.

However, a hair weave can place prolonged tension on thin hair, possibly causing damage and further hair loss. If considering a hair weave, make sure your hair can withstand the stress.

Hairpieces

These are hairnets, also called wiglets, woven with strands of real or synthetic hair and tailor-made to cover large patches of balding. With some hairpieces, natural hair can be pulled through for blending to build volume and height. Hairpieces come in assorted sizes, base material, and colors and can be dyed to match your natural hair color.

Human-hair wiglets are more expensive than synthetic hairpieces and can cost from $500 to $3,500. The better quality your hairpiece is, the less detectable it is when worn. About every six weeks, you may have to see your beautician for a service visit to have the hairpiece restyled or refitted. The cost of a service visit is $50 to $100 per visit.

There are many ways of attaching a hairpiece to your scalp. Some hairpieces are clipped or taped to your head. With clips, tiny fasteners are sewn right into the hairpiece. You simply clip the hairpiece onto your existing hairs. When you need bangs, clip-on hairpieces are great to wear under a hat. A downside of clips is that they can be uncomfortable.

Tape is the most convenient method of affixing a hairpiece to your scalp. A lot of tapes are waterproof now, so you can play sports or swim without worrying that your hairpiece will come off.

For greater permanence, other hairpieces are bonded on with special adhesives. Bonding is the most secure method of fastening a hairpiece to your scalp. Some of the terms for bonding include *megabond*, *polybond*, and *polyfuse*. After about four to six weeks, the bonding becomes loose, and you have to have new bonding materials applied by your hair replacement professional.

There are also hairpieces that are woven into your existing hair. You will want to choose the attachment that is the most secure for your needs.

Depending on how your hairpiece is attached, some must be removed each night, while others can be worn for as long as a month at a time. In addition, hairpieces need to be replaced periodically due to fading of hair in sunlight and general wear and tear. Synthetic hair is more durable and less subject to fading than human hair. Human hair, however, looks and feels more natural. On average, human hairpieces last about a year.

Another option is a type of hairpiece known as a "fall," a pony-tail-shaped piece of human or synthetic hair that can be used to add thickness and volume to thinning hair, or to form buns, chignons, or braids.

Wigs

Wigs date back to the fourth century B.C., to the ancient Egyptians, who shaved their heads to prevent insect infestation. Egyptian wigs were fashioned from palm and wood fibers, animal hair, even precious metals and secured to the scalp with beeswax. Since ancient times, wigs have evolved to become an important cosmetic adornment with a wide variety of uses.

Used to be, wigs were fuddy-duddy, fake-looking hats of hair. Not any more. New technologies in design and fit have made today's wigs indistinguishable from a real head of hair. The key is selecting a wig that fits your face and head and is professionally designed.

Wigs come in various sizes, or you can order a custom-fitted wig. Thus, when buying a wig, make sure the seller measures your head. That way, you'll get a better fit. Mail-order wig companies usually provide a step-by-step guide for self-measuring.

You can purchase wigs that are either styled or unstyled. Unstyled wigs have been cut, shaped, or curled. All you have to do is comb, brush, or pick them. Or you can go to a professional wig stylist for some extra finishing work.

A styled wig needs no styling on your part. It comes ready to wear. Just put it on—and voilà, you're ready to go.

Another advantage of wigs: You can own several and thus change your look to match your mood or the occasion, or make a complete personality change, depending on the situation.

Today, wigs are made of many different types of material: human hairs, synthetic hairs, and a blend of the two. Human hair wigs are designed with Chinese, Indonesian, and European hair, each with different characteristics. Indonesian hair, for example, is very fine, while Chinese hair is more coarse. European hair is strong and makes the most natural-looking of all human hair wigs.

Human hair wigs are very easy to style. They can be permed, blow-dried, even colored. Whatever you do to your own hair, you can do to a human hair wig. Generally, they last three to four years with proper care. However, if you dye a human hair wig, the hair fibers can weaken and break.

Wigs made of human and synthetic hair blended together can be permed and curled and are easy to care for. They generally last about two to three years.

Less expensive than human hair or blended wigs, synthetic hair wigs can't be permed, blow-dried, or colored. Nor do they feel as soft as human hair wigs. In terms of style, what you buy is generally what you wear. A synthetic wig will provide about one year of wear, depending on how you take care of it. Well-made synthetic hair wigs can look very natural. They hold curl very well and do not fade as fast as human hair wigs do.

When buying a wig, give some thought to color. Usually, you'll want to match the color of your present hair. Many companies will custom-dye wigs to match your natural color. Provide your wig supplier with a swatch of your own hair, or a sample hair color chosen from a hair-coloring product. If you don't have your wig custom-colored, examine the color swatches provided by various wig manufacturers to achieve the closest match.

Another important consideration when buying a wig is its cap. This is the part of the wig that fits directly on your scalp, and there are several types.

- Wefted wigs have pieces of hair sewn into the cap itself and look virtually capless.

- Mesh caps are made from very fine material in which individual hairs are woven by hand into nylon or polyester-based netting. Some mesh caps are coated with thin latex to create the illusion of a scalp with hair growing out of it.
- Vacuum caps provide an airtight seal on your scalp for a better fit. The cap is made from silicone that can be tinted to match the color of your skin. Wigs with vacuum caps fit so securely on your head that you can participate in sports or drive in a convertible without fear of the wig flying off. These wigs last two to three years.
- Hair integration caps feature openings that let you pull your existing hair through for a fuller, more natural look.

No matter what type or style of wig you purchase, be sure to follow the manufacturer's directions for proper care. Some manufacturers offer reconditioning services that clean, condition, and restyle your wig for a fee.

In addition, if you regularly wear a wig, don't neglect your scalp. Keeping it clean will help prevent irritation and further skin problems.

Also, if you're wearing a wig while your hair grows back after chemotherapy, make sure the wig fits properly. A poor fit exerts excessive pressure on parts of the scalp. The affected hair follicles may die, and your hair may not grow back. Specialists who work with cancer patients suggest choosing wigs that do not need to be affixed with glue, tape, or tight-fitting elastic bands.

Hats and Caps

Another option to consider is wearing a hat as a way to temporarily conceal thinning hair. Numerous companies make attractive hats, in various styles, expressly for women who have lost their hair due to chemotherapy, androgenetic alopecia, alopecia areata, or aging.

You can choose from turbans, short and long-brimmed hats, floppy-brimmed hats, sporty caps, halo hats, berets, headbands—

even hats with attached hair. For information on where to shop for a suitable hat, see Appendix B in the resource section under "Hats" on pages 226–228.

Newer Hair Systems

Numerous companies have introduced nonsurgical hair restoration technologies that provide viable, natural-looking alternatives to hair loss problems. These hair systems are made from ultra-thin, skinlike bases that are glued on to the scalp with a medical adhesive.

TRANSDERMAL HAIR RESTORATION (THR)

One of these newer systems is Transdermal Hair Restoration (THR), which offers a solution to hair loss without surgery. Introduced in 1996, THR features a transparent artificial skinlike membrane containing single strands of human hair matched to your own in color and texture. The membrane is so thin that if you touch it, you feel only hair and scalp.

With an FDA-approved bonding agent, this artificial graft is applied directly to the thinning areas of the scalp to cover patches of baldness and blend in with your existing hair. The graft is gas permeable, too, so your scalp can breathe and shed skin cells normally. THR works well for many types of hair loss, including alopecia areata, medically induced hair loss, and balding due to burns, accidents, or other trauma. If you want to check out THR for yourself, visit their website: www.emerging-solutions.com.

DERMAL RETENTION HAIR FILAMENT

Another new type of hair system is the Dermal Retention Hair Filament from United Micro Systems, Inc. This system consists of an ultra-fine fiber (the hair filament) in which individual hairs have been inserted. Unlike a hairpiece, there is no solid base, just a small circle of hairs attached to this filament.

In a procedure that takes several hours, these filaments are interblended with your own hair and adhered to the scalp with a special solution. As your own hair grows, it has to be trimmed to match the length of the artificial hair. Also, the system has to be removed monthly, cleaned, and put back on.

The average cost of the procedure is $2,000 to $8,500, depending on the degree of scalp coverage or hair length you desire. Promotional materials note that many television and movie stars have undergone the procedure, which gives results that are eight to ten times thicker than a hair transplant and without the surgical discomfort.

Dermal Retention is reversible and comes with a full lifetime warranty, but you have to travel to New Jersey to have it done. For more information, you can call the company toll-free at 1–800–235–5620, or e-mail at umsystem@voicenet.com. In addition, United Micro Systems, Inc. has a website explaining its procedure: www.unitedmicrosystems.com.

FOLLIGRAFT

Folligraft is another nonsurgical option featuring a porous membrane that resembles a layer of skin. The membrane is transparent so that it takes on the color of your skin. Before the Folligraft membrane is applied, your scalp is exfoliated to remove any dead skin cells. Next, the membrane is attached using medical-grade, FDA-approved bonding agents. Hair matching your own in color, texture, and curl is inserted into the membrane in a natural fashion. It looks and acts like real hair.

Folligraft is not a surgical procedure, so it does not require the services of a physician. However, only a certified, licensed Folligraft technician is allowed to perform it. For information on the procedure, its costs, and how to locate a licensed Folligraft professional, visit the company's website: www.folligraft.com.

Combinations

Increasingly, many women are opting for a partial surgical hair transplant and a partial hair system. Such a combination is a good alternative if you have a limited amount of donor hair but need more fullness. Wearing a natural-appearing partial hair system can help you achieve that look.

Also, since hair transplant surgery often takes from one to two years to complete, you might opt to temporarily wear a hair system while undergoing the procedure. That way, you won't have to appear in public looking as if your hair and scalp are undergoing surgery.

If you're among the unlucky ones who have suffered a bad hair transplant, wearing a hair system may be your best hope.

Locating a Qualified Hair Replacement Specialist

If you're considering a wig or other hair system, ask the potential supplier:

- How long have you been in business?
- What exchange and return policies do you offer?
- How much experience do your technicians have?
- Can I obtain references from your clients? Meeting with other clients is a great idea. That way, you can see how detectable their hair systems are, as well as learn whether these clients are happy with the supplier in question.

It's a good idea to check with your local Better Business Bureau to learn if any complaints have been lodged against the supplier you're considering. If several complaints have been registered, find another company.

A fairly recent development in the hair systems field is the new standard for Certified Replacement Specialists. This is a certification program for hair replacement professionals in which they take an American Hair Loss Council (AHLC) accredited course, fifty hours of specialty training, and twenty hours of continuing education every two years. In addition, a certified hair replacement professional must agree to a code of ethical behavior and be a member in good standing with the AHLC.

Try to find a hair replacement professional who has been

certified under this program. To locate a professional in your area, contact the AHLC (see Appendix B on page 222) and request the organization's *Source Book*. An experienced, certified specialist is your best bet for obtaining a hair system that looks natural and fits your lifestyle.

Epilogue:
Future Hair Savers

S CIENTISTS the world over are working earnestly on a true cure for baldness, and the good news is they're close. Within several years, expect to see a whole new arsenal of weapons to fight hair loss and baldness. What follows is a crystal-ball glimpse into the future of hair-saving technology:

Advanced Androgens and
5 Alpha-Reductase Inhibitors

Scientists are working on more ways to block the action of androgens so that hair follicles can begin sprouting hair again. Among the agents under investigation are:

- MK-0434. This drug has been found to inhibit follicle-damaging DHT by up to 95 percent. It works like finasteride—by inhibiting the enzyme 5 alpha-reductase, which converts testosterone to follicle-damaging DHT.
- MK-0963. Similarly, this drug, which is also a 5 alpha-reductase inhibitor, blocks DHT by 78 to 80 percent.
- MK-386. This antiandrogen inhibits 5 alpha-reductase type 1 only, and in experiments reduced the production of DHT by 89 percent when combined with finasteride.

- RU 58841. This drug is an androgen receptor blocker, meaning that it prevents androgens from latching onto their cellular receptors and entering cells. The drug inhibits the action of testosterone and DHT on hair follicles. Tested on monkeys, RU 58841 dramatically increased hair growth on the animals' frontal scalps.

There are fifteen or more other similar antibaldness agents currently under investigation throughout the world.

Aromatases

As I noted in Chapter Three, women have six times more follicle-protecting aromatase in their frontal scalp skin than men do. Aromatase is an enzyme that converts some testosterone and DHT into estrogen. Estrogen opposes the effects of testosterone and thus may help promote hair growth. Currently, aromatase is being investigated as an antiandrogen to treat androgenetic alopecia.

Beta-Catenin

Researchers at the University of Chicago's Howard Hughes Center have discovered a protein called *beta-catenin* that converts normal skin cells into hair follicles. A messenger molecule containing this protein was inserted into the skin cells of mice, and the cells transformed into hair follicle cells. With this discovery, it looks like new hair follicles can be regenerated, thus raising the possibility of a cure for baldness.

There is still much work to be done with animals before testing the protein on humans, especially since beta-catenin led to a high incidence of hair-follicle tumors. Scientists need to figure out how this protein is regulated inside the cell of the developing hair follicle before pursuing human studies.

Culturing Hair Matrix Cells

Scientists are working on culturing hair matrix cells to yield an unlimited supply of donor hair. At present, the work is being done on mice, but testing on humans is expected to begin in the near future. Basically, the cells are grown in the laboratory, then implanted into the scalp to grow hair.

Estrogen Blockers

In 1996, researchers at North Carolina State University in Raleigh accidentally discovered that an estrogen-blocking compound had the surprising side effect of reawakening dormant hair follicles.

The amazing discovery was made while scientists were studying how pesticides interact biochemically with estrogen. During these experiments, they noticed that hair stopped growing on the shaved coats of mice who had been treated topically with a certain type of estrogen called 17-beta estradiol. Then, after they applied an estrogen blocker called ICI 182,780 on the mice, the animals grew a full coat of hair in just four weeks. Somehow, the estrogen blocker signaled the hair follicles to regrow hair.

The scientists believe the estrogen blocker may stimulate hair growth in balding humans, too. If so, it could be a bona fide treatment for hair loss caused by chemotherapy and androgenetic alopecia. Studies on people will begin soon, but it could take several years or more before testing is completed and the treatment is commercially available.

Gene Therapy

In the very near future, it may be possible to rejuvenate gray hair and reactivate dormant hair follicles—all with gene therapy.

Quite by accident, scientists at AntiCancer, Inc., a small biotech company in San Diego, California, discovered a way to birth hair-producing skin cells. While growing cancer cells in the lab, they tried cultivating normal human skin cells and found that not only did the skin cells grow, they produced hair.

This serendipitous event led the scientists to further investigation. They found that they could transform skin cells into hair follicles by introducing a special gene into the hair follicle.

Scientists at AntiCancer, Inc. have already invented a way to deliver to the hair follicles the natural pigment that gives hair its color. Just imagine: Within several years, it may be possible to color your hair permanently—no more telltale roots.

Hair Cloning

Cloning—making exact replicas of hair like documents off a copy machine—may make it possible for you to have an unlimited crop of donor hair for a hair transplant. That way, a hair transplant surgeon can fill in your balding areas without worrying about how much hair is left at the donor site.

Experiments into hair cloning are being conducted in the United States and Great Britain.

Isoquinolines

Sunstar, Inc., of Japan manufactures Norreticuline and Reticuline, two drugs known as isoquinolines, which are opium alkaloids but do not have the narcotic effect or addiction potential. Both drugs appear to stimulate hair follicle cells in lab dishes. Norreticuline has activated hair growth in mice, and researchers believe the drugs could do the same in humans when applied topically. But how the drugs work to grow hair has not been investigated in detail.

Minoxidil-Like Medicines

The success of minoxidil as a hair-restorer has led scientists to examine other drugs that are used in the treatment of hypertension. Among those that grow hair when applied topically are pinacidil, cromakalim, and diazoxide.

In experiments with monkeys, diazoxide (applied topically) thickened hair, enlarged the hair follicles, and accelerated the hair-growing cycle from telogen to anagen. Apparently, testing on the drug's hair-growing benefits are under way. As an oral medication diazoxide has numerous side effects, including serious heart problems.

None of these drugs has been officially approved to treat hair loss.

Parathyroid Hormone Related
Peptide (PTHrP) Antagonist

PTHrP is a chemical made by skin cells that causes hair follicles to enter their resting stage. Led by Michael Holick, M.D., scientists at Boston University believe that by blocking this chemical with a PTHrP antagonist, hair follicles can start growing hair again. In fact, tests on mice revealed that the antagonist stimulated hair growth in 100 percent of the follicles. Blocking the action of PTHrP with an antagonist keeps follicles from going to sleep, and they continue to grow hair.

Experiments with people are now under way. If those tests are successful, a treatment could be available in five years. The PTHrP antagonist looks very promising.

And Finally . . .

Saving your hair isn't something that happens overnight. It can take months and years to stop or reverse the shedding, and even then there are no guarantees. With the approval of your dermatologist, be willing to experiment and try different combinations of treatments: diet, medications, and supplements, for example. Often, it's the most comprehensive approach that works best, but it takes some trial and error—and a huge dose of patience! Once you find what works best for you, stick with it.

Through all of this, remember that you're more than a head of hair. You have been blessed with unique qualities and gifts that add up to so much more than how you look in the mirror. True beauty is a reflection not of what's on the outside but of what's on the inside.

Glossary

General Terminology

5 Alpha-Reductase: Enzymes that convert the hormone testosterone to dihydrotestosterone (DHT), the hormone that damages hair follicles in people suffering from androgenetic alopecia. There are two forms of these enzymes, type 1 and type 2.

Alopecia: Medical term for baldness.

Alopecia areata: The medical term for patchy hair loss on the scalp. Alopecia areata is believed to be caused by a disorder of the immune system.

Alopecia totalis: A form of alopecia areata in which hair is lost from the entire scalp.

Alopecia universalis: A form of alopecia areata in which hair is lost over the entire body.

Amino acids: The building blocks of protein. A deficiency of amino acids may adversely affect hair growth.

Anagen: The growing phase of the hair cycle.

Anagen effluvium: Hair loss caused by chemotherapeutic drugs.

Androgenetic alopecia: Hair loss resulting from a genetic predisposition to effects of DHT on the hair follicles. Also termed *female-pattern baldness* and *male-pattern baldness*.

Androgens: Male hormones such as testosterone and DHT.

Antiandrogen: An agent that blocks the action of androgens by preventing their attachment to receptors on cells, interfering with their metabolism, or decreasing their production in the body.

Aromatase: An enzyme present in the root of the follicle that plays a protective role against androgenetic alopecia.

Azelaic acid: A medication used to treat acne. Azelaic acid inhibits the activity of the enzyme 5 alpha-reductase, involved in the conversion of testosterone to DHT.

Catagen: The transitional phase of the hair cycle occurring after anagen and before telogen.

Club hair: Hair that sits in the resting follicle.

Cortex: The main structural part of the hair fiber.

Cuticle: The outermost portion of the hair fiber.

Cyproterone acetate (CPA): An antiandrogen drug used to treat androgenetic alopecia in women. It is not available in the United States.

Dermal papilla: A structure at the base of the hair follicle. It is rich in blood vessels that supply nutrients to construct keratin.

Dihydrotestosterone (DHT): A hormone formed when the enzyme 5 alpha-reductase interacts with testosterone. DHT is believed to destroy hair follicles in androgenetic alopecia.

Finasteride: The generic name for the drugs Propecia and Proscar. Finasteride works by blocking 5 alpha-reductase, an enzyme required to convert testosterone into DHT.

Follicle: A sacklike structure just below the surface of your scalp. Hair grows from the follicle.

Gene therapy: An experimental method of inserting a special gene into the hair follicle to stimulate hair growth.

Keratin: A tough but elastic protein from which hair is constructed.

Ketoconazole: An antifungal agent that has antiandrogenetic properties.

Lanugo: The fine, soft, colorless hair covering a fetus and shed at about the eighth month of fetal development.

Medulla: The innermost portion of the hair fiber.

Melanocytes: Cells that produce the pigment which determines hair color.

Miniaturization: The destructive process by which DHT shrinks hair follicles and causes them to deteriorate over time, thus triggering hair loss.

Minoxidil: The generic name for the drug Rogaine or other products, approved for treating hair loss in men and women. Minoxidil is available as an over-the-counter drug in a 2 percent solution, as well as a prescription drug in a 5 percent concentration.

Nonscarring alopecia: A broad category of different types of hair loss, including androgenetic alopecia. In nonscarring alopecia, the hair follicle remains intact, thus increasing the likelihood that hair loss can be reversed.

Nonvellus hair: Hairs that are thick and dark. Normal scalp hair is considered nonvellus hair. Also called *terminal hair*.

Retin-A: A brand name for a prescription acne medication. Retin-A has been shown to be effective against hair loss, particularly when combined with minoxidil.

Saw palmetto: An herb with antiandrogen properties.

Scarring alopecia: Patchy hair loss with obvious signs of scalp inflammation.

Sebum: An oily secretion manufactured by tiny sebaceous glands near the follicles that keeps your hair lubricated and shiny.

Spironolactone: A diuretic drug that acts as an antiandrogen.

Telogen: The resting phase of the hair cycle.

Telogen effluvium: The second most common form of hair loss. It is usually the result of severe stress, illness, major surgery, childbirth, and the use of certain medications. Telogen effluvium can be *delayed* (occurring a few months after the stressful incident) or *chronic* (unresolved).

Terminal hair: The coarser, pigmented hair that appears on the scalp, face, armpits, and pubic areas. Also called *nonvellus hair*.

Testosterone: A male hormone that promotes the development of male characteristics.

Traction alopecia: Hair loss caused by tightly pulled hair styles.

Trichotillomania: Habitual hair-pulling.

Vellus: The soft, fluffy postnatal hair that remains on the entire body, except for the palms of the hands, soles of the feet, and other normally hairless portions.

Hair Replacement Terminology

Dilator: A tiny, strawlike pin inserted into slits or holes to widen them.

Donor site: An area of skin with healthy hair follicles that is surgically transplanted onto bald patches.

Flap: A type of hair replacement surgery in which a piece of hair-bearing scalp is cut on three or four sides and transplanted onto bald areas of the scalp.

Follicular units: Natural groupings of hairs that grow from the scalp.

Follicular unit transplantation: An advanced form of hair transplantation in which the surgeon harvests hair in naturally occurring follicular units and grafts them to balding sections of your scalp.

Grafting: A variety of procedures describing the removal of hair-bearing scalp from the back of the head to a recipient site. The most widely used types of grafting are slit grafts, micrografting, and minigrafting.

Grafts: Transplanted hair.

Linear graft: A row of hair and skin that is transplanted onto bald regions.

Micrograft: A grouping of one to three hairs used in a hair transplant and inserted into needle holes.

Minigraft: Small rectangles or circles of three to eight follicles each.

Punch graft: A group of ten to twenty hairs in a circular graft.

Recipient site: A bald area of the scalp onto which hair grafts are transplanted.

Scalp reduction: A procedure that involves the surgical removal of a strip of hairless scalp to reduce the total area of baldness. Then, the remainder is pulled together and sutured closed. This reduces the bald area.

Slit graft: A graft of three to four hairs inserted into a slit rather than a round hole.

Soft tissue expansion: A type of scalp reduction surgery in which balloons are inserted under the hair-bearing area of the scalp to stretch it. Next, the bags are removed, and the bald area of the scalp is cut out. Flaps are created from the expanded hair-bearing skin.

Resources

For additional information, look to support groups and medical associations. These organizations are among the best authorities for detailed and up-to-date information to help you cope with your situation. Support groups, in particular, devote themselves to disseminating information to those who need it. Here are key organizations that can provide you with additional information on hair loss.

Professional Organizations

American Academy of Cosmetic Surgery (AACS)
401 North Michigan Avenue
Chicago, IL 60611
312–527-6713 or 800-A-NEW-YOU (263–9968)
312–644-1815 (fax)
www.cosmeticsurgeryonline.com

The AACS is a leading organization of practitioners in various medical disciplines, including dermatology, plastic and reconstructive surgery, general surgery, and cosmetic dentistry, among others. It is the nation's largest organization representing board-certified cosmetic surgeons. The AACS website provides a surgeon search, information on procedures, an article archive, and other items of interest.

A specialty subgroup of the AACS is the American Society of Hair Restoration Surgery (ASHRS) (see page 222).

American Academy of Dermatology
930 North Meacham Road
Schaumburg, IL 60173–6016
847–330-0230 or 888–462-DERM (462–3376)
www.aad.org

The AAD was founded in 1938 and is today the largest and most influential dermatologic association. With more than eleven thousand members, it is the certifying body for physicians who wish to be certified in dermatology. The organization is committed to advancing the science and art of medicine and surgery related to the skin; promoting high standards in clinical practice, education, and research in dermatology; supporting and enhancing patient care; and promoting the public interest relating to dermatology through public education programs.

American Academy of Plastic
& Reconstruction Surgeons (ASPRS)
444 East Algonquin Road
Arlington Heights, IL 60005
847–228-9900
www.plasticsurgery.org

The ASPRS is a professional association of plastic surgeons. On its website, you can find information on hair restoration surgery and locate a surgeon by name or geographical area.

American Board of Hair Restoration
Surgery (ABHRS)
18525 South Torrence Avenue
Lansing, IL 60438
708–474-2600

Founded in 1996, the ABHRS certifies surgeons in the hair restoration field. Its mission is to improve the quality of patient care by giving patients an objective way to judge the qualifications of physicians who practice hair restoration. The organization advises patients considering hair transplants to ask surgeons if they are certified by the ABHRS.

American Hair Loss Council
401 North Michigan Avenue
Chicago, IL 60611
312–321-5128
312–245-1080 (fax)
www.ahlc.org

The AHLC is a nonprofit group that provides the public with non-biased information on treatments and options for hair loss. AHLS members are specialists who work with diagnosing, treating, and researching hair loss.

American Society for Dermatologic Surgery (ASDS)
800–441-2737
www.asda-net.org

Founded in 1970, the ASDS is an organization for dermatologists that promotes excellence in the specialty and fosters high standards of patient care. It supports research, provides continuing education for its members, and sponsors community outreach programs for the public.

American Society of Hair Restoration Surgery (ASHRS)
401 North Michigan Avenue
Chicago, IL 60611–4267
312–527-6713
312–644-1815 (fax)

A specialty subgroup of the American Academy of Cosmetic Surgery, the ASHRS fosters the growth and quality of practice of hair restoration surgery worldwide through the exchange of information among surgeons. The organization also supports the development of new standards and research in the field.

International Society of Hair Restoration Surgery (ISHRS)
930 North Meacham Road
Schaumburg, IL 60173–6016
847–330-9830 or 800–444-2737
847–330-1135 (fax)
www.ishrs.org

The ISHRS is a professional organization of hair restoration surgeons. The organization's website offers information on hair restoration as well as a "physician finder" to help you locate a surgeon in your area.

Support Organizations

National Alopecia Areata Foundation (NAAF)
710 C Street, Suite 11
San Rafael, CA 94901–3853
415-456–4644

Established in 1981, the NAAF is a national support organization for people with alopecia areata. Its mission is to disseminate information about the disease, raise funds for research, and provide valuable information to sufferers. The organization can also provide the names of local support groups in your geographical area.

Trichotillomania Learning Center, Inc. (TLC)
1215 Mission Street, Suite 2
Santa Cruz, CA 95060
408-457–1004
www.trich.org

Founded in 1991, TLC is a national nonprofit organization dedicated to advancing the understanding of trichotillomania (compulsive hair pulling). TLC's website provides information on where to find support groups in your geographical area. It also provides information on treatment options for trichotillomania.

Recommended Reading

The Bald Truth: The First Complete Guide to Preventing and Treating Hair Loss
Spencer David Kobren
(Pocket Books, 1998)

Spencer David Kobren is a consumer activist with a radio show called "The Bald Truth." Even though this book is written for men, it contains an excellent discussion and understandable overview of various hair restoration procedures. The book also clearly explains the role androgens play in triggering hair loss. Easy to read, this book will enlighten you on many issues relating to hair loss.

Hair Loss Treatment Almanac 1998
David Tse
(TSE Publishing, 1997)

This book is an excellent review of prescription, nonprescription, and alternative treatments for hair-loss sufferers. It is very informative and helpful, with phone numbers and addresses of various hair care product suppliers. For information on ordering this book, contact TSE Publishing, Inc., 163 Third Avenue, Suite 300, New York, NY 10003; or order it from the Internet bookstore, www.amazon.com.

Hair Loss Prevention Through Natural Remedies
Ken Peters, David Stuss, and Nick Waddell
(Apple Publishing Company, Ltd., 1996)

If you want to further explore the role natural remedies can play in hair-loss prevention, this book is an excellent resource. It covers vitamins, minerals, essential fatty acids, herbs, juices, and other dietary issues. You'll learn a lot about the benefits of these approaches by reading this book.

Hair: An Owner's Manual
Philip Kingsley
(Aurum, 1995)

Author Philip Kingsley is a well-known expert on hair. For an excellent look at how to take care of your hair, you'll want this book in your library.

Websites

www.baldness.net: This website links you to other hair loss resources on the Internet. You'll find links to general baldness information, baldness treatments, newsgroups, clinics, and centers—even sites featuring baldness humor.

www.follicle.com: If you're looking for information on different types of treatment, you'll find it here. This site covers in detail the specifics of drug and nondrug treatments for all types of hair loss.

www.hairloss.com: This site brings together up-to-date information on hair loss, its causes, and various treatments available. It can also put you in touch with hair-loss experts in the United States and Canada. And you'll find links to other hair-loss sites of interest.

www.hairsite.com: This website provides easy-to-read profiles of hair-loss products currently being marketed, with information on how to order them. Also, there is a lively message forum in which you can cyberchat with other hair-loss sufferers and find out what has worked and not worked for them.

www.hairtoday.com: This website features interview transcripts of chats with hair-loss experts. It also has a "hair store" from which you can purchase assorted products. A message board lets you post questions to others who visit the site. Each month, there are updates on current developments in the care and treatment of baldness.

www.keratin.com: This very comprehensive site provides information on hair, hair disorders, and treatment. There are numerous sections that can link you to resources for your particular case.

www.morehair.com: Here you'll find information about hair growth, hair loss, surgery, drugs, supplements, and nutrition.

www.nerdworld.com: Simply type in the word *hair* into this site's search engine, and you'll be transported to a list of links on hair-loss prevention, hair replacement, and hair care.

www.regrowth.com: This excellent site contains updated information on every form of hair-loss treatment that exists, from nondrug approaches to the latest in hair transplant techniques. Reports and findings from medical conventions are here, too. In addition, there are regular interviews with the world's leading hair-loss experts. Be sure to check out the section titled "Hair Loss Sites." It features more than two hundred links to commercial and noncommercial hair-loss sites. Regrowth.com is a handy resource.

www.stayhealthy.com: Input the word *alopecia* in the site's search engine, and a list of resources and links will appear.

Hats

ESPECIALLY FOR YOU BY SUSIE Q
This company has many different styles of hats and turbans—all machine washable. For more information, visit its website: www.susieqcreations.com.

HAT AND SOUL
Hat and Soul was founded on a friendship. Two women who shared a love of sewing and a love of hats were inspired to create a hat company after another friend, undergoing chemotherapy, had no options for concealing her hair loss. Hat and Soul was born.

This company offers some truly beautiful and elegant hats—hats any woman would love to wear—and there are several styles from which to choose. Contact Hat and Soul at: www.hatandsoul.com.

HEADCOVERS UNLIMITED

This company offers hats, wigs, and turbans for women experiencing hair loss. The products are quite fashionable—and elegant. Contact Headcovers Unlimited at its website: www.head covers.com.

HIP HAT

Hip Hats are hats with hairpieces. The company offers nine styles of hats, fifteen colors of hair, and four different hair textures. The hats and hair are sold separately. The company's website is: www.hip-hat.com.

JUST IN TIME

Headquartered in Philadelphia, Pennsylvania, this company was founded by Verley Platt, who suffered hair loss as a result of chemotherapy for breast cancer. During that time, she could not find any suitable headwear to conceal her balding pate. After completing treatment, she began designing hats that are well made, flattering, and fun to wear. Just in Time offers a wide range of turban-style hats. For more information, contact the company at: P.O. Box 27506, Philadelphia, PA 19118, 215–247-8777; or visit the company's website: www.softhats.com.

TWO WOMEN WITH HATS

The founder of Two Women with Hats, Carol Sanchez, is a certified breast and lymphedema compression garment fitter and a custom breast fitter/personal consultant. She created the company to help women with cancer cope with hair loss by providing a selection of attractive headwear. Her daughter Christine works with her in managing the company.

The products offered are among the most fashionable you'll

find, from stylish brimmed hats to berets to attractive turbans. Check out the selections at: www.womenhats.com.

VP DESIGNS

This company makes "halo hats," a two piece-construction of a doughnut-shaped halo and the fitted skull cap. It is a very attractive design and comes in a variety of patterns and colors. You can order halo hats through: www.shopbuilder.com.

Purchasing Hair Care Products and Medicines

As you learn more about hair-loss treatments, you're bound to run across some dubious products. Many fraudulent products, including those for baldness, are being promoted by unscrupulous marketers.

How can you recognize a fraud? According to the FDA, the warning signs of a fraudulent marketer are:

- The product is described as having a "secret formula."
- The product claims to be a miracle cure and/or provides easy, dramatic results.
- Testimonials and anecdotes are used to support claims.

If you feel a fraudulent marketer has duped you, there is recourse. Contact one of these organizations:

- FDA, Consumer Affairs and Information, 5600 Fishers Lane, HFC-110, Rockville, MD 20857 (or look for your local FDA listing in the telephone directory under the United States Department of Health and Human Services).
- Your state's Attorney General's Office.
- The Federal Trade Commission (FTC), Correspondence Branch, Room 692, Sixth and Pennsylvania Avenues, N.W., Washington, D.C. 20260.
- The U.S. Postal Service Chief Postal Inspector, 475 L'Enfant Plaza, Washington, D.C. 20260 (or your local postmaster)— for fraudulent or quack products ordered by mail.

Purchasing Hair Care Products
Over the Internet

With the click of a computer mouse—and without even seeing a doctor—you can purchase prescription medications, including hair-loss drugs, over the Internet. Case in point: Propecia, a prescription drug approved for men's baldness, is sold through various Internet sites, and no prescription is needed. Further, many drugs marketed via the Internet are not approved for sale in the United States.

In most instances, websites that sell medicines pass orders on to pharmacies that have agreed to process orders for them, provided the medicine is not a controlled substance such as a narcotic.

This book has discussed a number of prescription medications for hair loss that are not yet available in the United States but are fairly common elsewhere in the world. Some of these drugs are sold through websites, and it's tempting to buy them. But if you're going to do so, talk to your personal physician or dermatologist first.

There's the chance that unapproved drugs, especially those available overseas, may have been produced under unknown or questionable manufacturing conditions, according to the FDA. Such products carry an increased risk of contamination, have questionable potency, and lack quality assurance, thus posing a potential hazard to the public.

Already, several states, in concert with the FDA, have begun investigating websites that engage in selling medicines in cyberspace. Some websites have been ordered to stop this practice unless patients have prescriptions from their physicians. In the near future, look for strict governmental regulation of on-line medicine peddling.

For your own health and well-being, don't experiment with any hair-loss drug, or purchase it from a website, unless your doctor has prescribed it for you and outlined its risks and side effects.

Importing Pharmaceuticals for Personal Use

As noted, some hair-loss medications are not approved for use in the United States, yet they have been used successfully for many years in Europe and other regions of the world. For a long time now, the FDA has let people import small quantities of foreign drugs for personal use—drugs that are unapproved for use in the United States. The policy applies to drugs carried in personal baggage or purchased through mail order. However, there are certain restrictions:

- The drug does not pose unreasonable or significant safety risks.
- Personal-use quantities are amounts designed for treatment of three months or less.
- The drug is not intended for commercial use. In other words, you can't resell it.
- The drug is designed to treat a serious condition in which there's no satisfactory treatment available in the United States.
- The imported drugs can't be a controlled substance (such as narcotics) or anabolic steroids.
- You must confirm in writing that you are using the drug under the supervision of a physician. The FDA has publicly stated that no one's well-being is served by having access to a drug for a serious disease without the active oversight of a licensed physician.

Despite this policy, be aware that buying and using prescription drugs without the help of a physician or other licensed health professional may violate state and local laws. Further, all drugs and cosmetics are subject to examination by the FDA when they arrive in the United States. And the FDA warns consumers that severe adverse reactions, including death, can result from the improper use of prescription drugs.

If you have questions about importing drugs for personal use, contact your local FDA district office or the Imports Operations Branch in Rockville, Maryland, at 301-443–6553.

References

A portion of the information in this book comes from medical research reports in both the popular and scientific publications, professional textbooks and booklets, promotional literature from hair care companies, Internet sources, and computer searches of medical databases of research abstracts.

Chapter One

Brown, C. V. 1997. "Examining Your Physician: Thoughts on Choosing Your Primary Care Provider." *The Network News*, November-December, 1–13.

Condor, B. 1998. "Americans Increasingly Trying Alternative Medicine, Study Shows." Knight-Ridder News Service, November 11, K2370.

Editor. 1999. "Alternative Health Care on the Rise." *Nutritional Outlook*, January-February, 12.

Editor. 1994. "Between Patient and Doctor." *Harvard Health Letter*, April, 9–12.

Editor. 1998. "Considering Alternative Medicine: How to Discuss Your Decision with Your Doctor." *Tufts University Health & Nutrition Letter*, November, 4-5.

Leviton, R. 1992. "Choosing the Right Practitioner." *Vegetarian Times*, September, 28–33.

Rauber, C. 1998. "Open to Alternatives: Pressured by Consumer Demand, More Health Plans Are Embracing Nontraditional Treatment Options." *Modern Healthcare*, September 7, 50.

Chapter Two

Aufderheide, J. 1989. "Your Hair's Growth Cycle." *Total Health*, February, 50–51.

Bisacre, M., R. Carlisle, D. Robertson, and J. Ruck. 1984. *The Illustrated Encyclopedia of the Human Body*. New York: Exeter Books.

Bonnichsen, R., and A. L. Schneider. 1995. "Roots." *The Sciences*, May-June, 26–31.

Courtois, M., G. Loussouarn, S. Hourseau, and J. F. Grollier. 1996. "Periodicity in the Growth and Shedding of Hair." *British Journal of Dermatology* 134: 47–54.

Dawber, R. 1988. "The Embryology and Development of Human Scalp Hair." *Clinics of Dermatology* 6: 1-6.

Editor. 1988. "Hair, Beautiful Hair." *Health News*, August, 1-5.

Henig, R. M. 1985. *How a Woman Ages*. New York: Ballantine Books.

Kaufman, M. 1998. "The Psychology of Hair." *Health*, July-August, 86–89.

Parkinson, R. W. 1992. "Hair Loss in Women: What to Say and Do to Ease These Patients' Distress." *Postgraduate Medicine* 91: 417–22.

Pine, D. 1991. "Hair! From Personal Statement to Personal Problem." *FDA Consumer*, December, 20–23.

Spindler, J. R., and J. L. Data. 1992. "Female Androgenetic Alopecia: A Review." *Dermatology Nursing* 4: 93–99.

Weiss, R. 1991. "Fuzzy Science: Researchers Brush Up on the Biology of Hair." *Science News*, March 16, 168–70.

Zuidema, G. 1986. *The John Hopkins Atlas of Human Functional Anatomy*. 3rd ed. Baltimore: The John Hopkins University Press.

Chapter Three

American Academy of Dermatology. 1996. "Guidelines of Care for Androgenetic Alopecia." *Journal of the American Academy of Dermatology* 35: 465–69.

———. 1998. "Hair Diseases in African-Americans Require Specialized Knowledge." ADA press release.

American Psychiatric Association. 1994. *Diagnostic and Statistical Manual of Mental Disorders: DSM-IV* 4th ed. American Psychiatric Association: Washington, D.C.

Barth, J. H. 1988. "Alopecia and Hirsutes—Current Concepts in Pathogenesis and Management." *Drugs* 35: 83–91.

Bergfeld, W. F. 1978. "Diffuse Hair Loss in Women." *Cutis* 22: 190–95.

Brodlund, D. G., and S. A. Muller. 1991. "Androgenetic Alopecia (Common Baldness)." *Cutis* 47: 173–76.

Dawber, R. P. R. 1981. "Common Baldness in Women." *International Journal of Dermatology* 20: 647–50.

Dawber, R. P. R., and B. L. Connor. 1971. "Pregnancy, Hair Loss, and the Pill." *British Medical Journal* 4: 234.

Editor. 1994. "The Latest on Baldness Cures." *Health News*, December, 4-6.

Editor. 1996. "What If Your Hair Falls Out in Patches?" *Executive Health's Good Health Report*, October, 7.

Federal Drug Administration. 1994. "FDA Warns Against Use of 'Rio' Hair Relaxer." FDA press release.

Fiedler, V. C., and S. Alaiti. 1996. "Treatment of Alopecia Areata." *Dermatologic Clinics* 14: 733–38.

Graedon, J., and T. Graedon. 1989. "Common Drugs Cause Hair Loss." *Medical SelfCare*, November-December, 23.

Grimalt, R., F. Ferrando, and F. Grimalt. 1998. "Trichodynia." *Dermatology* 196: 374.

Headington, J. T. 1993. "Telogen Effluvium." *Archives of Dermatology* 129: 356–63.

INK Electronic Media Limited. 1998. "Alopecia Info & Resources." Internet website: www.follicle.com.

Intrator, N. 1996. "The Terror of Hair Loss—Can You Make the Shedding Stop?" *Cosmopolitan*, December, 136–37.

Klaber, M. R., and D. D. Munro. 1974. "Hair and Its Problems." *Nursing Mirror and Midwives Journal* 139: 48–50.

Larson, D. E. 1990. *Mayo Clinic Family Health Book*. New York: William Morrow and Company, Inc.

Lebwohl, M. 1997. "New Treatments for Alopecia Areata." *Lancet* 349: 222–23.

Meisler, J. D. 1998. "Conversation with the Experts—Toward Optimal Health: The Experts Respond to Hair Loss in Women." *Journal of Women's Health* 7: 307–10.

Mortimer, P. S., and R. P. R. Dawber. 1984. "Hair Loss and Lithium." *International Journal of Dermatology* 20: 603–604.

Nicholson, A. G., C. C. Harland, R. H. Bull, et al. 1993. "Chemically Induced Cosmetic Alopecia." *British Journal of Dermatology* 128: 537–41.

Nielsen, T. A., and R. Martin. 1995. "Alopecia: Diagnosis and Management." *American Family Physician* 51: 1513–24.

Parkinson, R. W. 1992. "Hair Loss in Women—What to Say and Do to Ease These Patients' Distress." *Postgraduate Medicine* 91: 417–22.

Rapaport, J., and B. M. Rubin. 1997. "Are You Losing Your Hair?" *Good Housekeeping*, July, 41–43.

Rebora, A. 1997. "Telogen Effluvium." *Dermatology* 195: 209–12.

———. 1998a. "Trichodynia." *Dermatology* 196: 374.

———. 1998b. "Reply." *Dermatology* 196: 375.

Ro, B. I. 1995. "Alopecia Areata in Korea (1982–1994)." *Journal of Dermatology* 22: 858–64.

Roberts, J. L. 1997. "Androgenetic Alopecia in Men and Women; an Overview of Cause and Treatment." *Dermatology Nursing* 9: 379–88.

Rubin, M. B. 1997. "Androgenetic Alopecia—Battling a Losing Proposition." *Postgraduate Medicine* 2: 129–31.

Rushton, D. H., and M. J. Morris. 1992. "Hair Loss in Women." *Cosmetics and Toiletries*, November, 49–52.

Sahelian, R. 1998. "DHEA: The Promise of Hormones." *Better Nutrition*, May, 58–61.

Sawaya, M. E. 1994. "Biochemical Mechanisms Regulating Human Hair Growth." *Skin Pharmacology* 7: 5-7.

Setterberg, R. 1989. "Battle of the Bald." *Hippocrates*, September-October, 28–29.

Shapiro, J., and V. Price. 1998. "Hair Regrowth—Therapeutic Agents." *Dermatologic Clinics* 16: 341–56.

Soriana, J. L., R. L. O'Sullivan, L. Baer, et al. 1996. "Trichotillomania and Self-Esteem: A Survey of 62 Female Hair Pullers." *Journal of Clinical Psychiatry* 57: 77–82.

Sperling, L. C. and D. C. Mezebiah. 1998. "Hair Diseases." *Medical Clinics of North America* 82: 1155–59.

Steck, W. D. 1978. "Telogen Effluvium—a Clinically Useful Concept, with Traction Alopecia as an Example." *Cutis* 21: 543–48.

Trueb, R. M. 1995. "'Chignon alopecia': A Distinctive Type of Nonmarginal Traction Alopecia." *Cutis* 55: 178–79.

Van Neste, D. J. J., and D. H. Rushton. 1997. "Hair Problems in Women." *Clinics in Dermatology* 15: 113–25.

Venning, V. A. and R. P. R. Dawber. 1988. "Patterned Androgenetic Alopecia in Women." *Journal of the American Academy of Dermatology* 18: 1073–77.

Weitzner, J. M. 1990. "Alopecia Areata." *American Family Physician* 41: 1197–1201.

Whiting, D. A. 1996. "Chronic Telogen Effluvium: Increased Scalp Hair Shedding in Middle-Aged Women." *Journal of the American Academy of Dermatology* 35: 899–906.

———. 1996. "Chronic Telogen Effluvium." *Dermatologic Clinics* 14: 723–31.

Wygledowska-Kania, M., and T. Bogdanowski. 1995. "Testing the Significance of Psychic Factors in the Etiology of Alopecia Areata." Examination of Personality by Means of Eysenck's Personality Inventory (MPI) Adapted by Choynowski." *Przeglad Lekarski* 52: 562–64.

Chapter Four

Hordinsky, M. 1998. "Alopecia Areata." Internet website: www.npntserver. mcg.edu/htm/alopecia/documents/AAconcept.html.

Meisler, J. D. 1998. "Conversation with the Experts—Toward Optimal Health: The Experts Respond to Hair Loss in Women." *Journal of Women's Health* 7: 307–10.

Nielsen, T. A., and R. Martin. 1995. "Alopecia: Diagnosis and Management." *American Family Physician* 51: 1513–24.

Parkinson, R. W. 1992. "Hair Loss in Women—What to Say and Do to Ease These Patients' Distress." *Postgraduate Medicine* 91: 417–22.

Rushton, D. H., and M. J. Morris. 1992. "Hair Loss in Women." *Cosmetics and Toiletries*, November, 49–52.

Sperling, L. C., and D. C. Mezebiah. 1998. "Hair Diseases." *Medical Clinics of North America* 82: 1155–59.

Antibalding Medications

ANTHRALIN (MICANOL, DRITHOCREME, DRITHRO-SCALP)

Fiedler-Weiss, V. C., and C. M. Buys. 1987. "Evaluation of Anthralin in the Treatment of Alopecia Areata." *Archives of Dermatology* 123: 1491–93.

Fiedler, V. C., A. Wendrow, G. J. Szpunar, and R. L. DeVillez. 1990. "Treatment-Resistant Alopecia Areata. Response to Combination Therapy with Minoxidil Plus Anthralin." *Archives of Dermatology* 126: 756–59.

Editor. 1999. *Physicians' Desk Reference*. Montvale, N.J.: Medical Economics Company Inc.

AZELAIC ACID (AZELEX)

Editor. 1998. "Azelaic Acid." Internet website: www.follicle.com.

CIMETIDINE (TAGAMENT)

Aram, H. 1987. "Treatment of Female Androgenetic Alopecia with Cimetidine." *International Journal of Dermatology* 26: 128–30.

Editor. 1999. *Physicians' Desk Reference*. Montvale, N.J.: Medical Economics Company, Inc.

Editor. 1993. *The PDR Family Guide to Prescription Drugs*. Montvale, N.J.: Medical Economics Data, Inc.

CORTICOSTEROIDS

Editor. 1991. "Cortisone: The Limits of a 'Miracle.'" *Nutrition Health Review*, Fall, 12–13.

Editor. 1999. *Physicians' Desk Reference*. Montvale, N.J.: Medical Economics Company, Inc.

Editor. 1993. *The PDR Family Guide to Prescription Drugs*. Montvale, N.J.: Medical Economics Data, Inc.

Fisher, D. A. 1977. "Systemic Steroids for Treatment of Alopecia Areata." *Archives of Dermatology* 113: 1731–32.

Olsen, E. A., S. C. Carson, and E. A. Turney. 1992. "Systemic Steroids With or

Without 2% Topical Minoxidil in the Treatment of Alopecia Areata. *Archives of Dermatology* 128: 1467–73.

Sharma, V. K. 1996. "Pulsed Administration of Corticosteroids in the Treatment of Alopecia Areata." *International Journal of Dermatology* 35: 133–36.

Zoorob, R. J., and D. Cender. 1998. "A Different Look at Corticosteroids." *American Family Physician* 58: 443–50.

CYPROTERONE ACETATE (ANDROCUR)

Blanchard, G., and B. Blanchard. 1989. "Approach to Hair Loss Reduction." *Journal of the National Medical Association* 81: 755–56.

Callan, A. W., and J. Montalto. 1995. "Female Androgenetic Alopecia: An Update." *Australasian Journal of Dermatology* 36: 51–55.

Diamanti-Kandarakis, E., G. Tolis, and A. J. Duleba. 1995. "Androgens and Therapeutic Aspects of Antiandrogens in Women." *Journal of the Society for Gynecologic Investigation* 2: 577–92.

Ekoe, J. M., P. Burchhardt, and B. Ruedi. 1980. "Treatment of Hirsutism, Acne and Alopecia with Cyproterone Acetate." *Dermatologica* 160: 398–404.

Mortimer, C. H., H. Rushton, and K. C. James. 1984. "Effective Medical Treatment for Common Baldness in Women." *Clinical and Experimental Dermatology* 9: 342–50.

Nardi, M., D. De Aloysio, P. Busacchi, and C. Flamigni. 1975. "Cyproterone Acetate—Ethinyl Estradiol Treatment of Hirsutism, Acne, Seborrhea and Alopecia." *Acta Europaea Fertilitatis* 6: 153–65.

Peereboom-Wynia, J. D., A. H. Van der Willigen, T. Van Joost, and E. Stolz. 1989. "The Effect of Cyproterone Acetate on Hair Roots and Hair Shaft Diameter in Androgenetic Alopecia in Females." *Acta Dermato-Venereologica* 69: 395–98.

Rushton, D. H. 1993. "Management of Hair Loss in Women." *Dermatologic Clinics* 11: 47–53.

Rushton, D. H., and I. D. Ramsey. 1992. "The Importance of Adequate Serum Ferritin Levels During Oral Cyproterone Acetate and Ethinyl Estradiol Treatment of Diffuse Androgen-Dependent Alopecia in Women." *Clinical Endocrinology* 36: 421–27.

ESTROGEN

Editor. 1999. *Physicians' Desk Reference*. Montvale, N.J.: Medical Economics Company, Inc.

Editor. 1993. *The PDR Family Guide to Prescription Drugs*. Montvale, N.J.: Medical Economics Data, Inc.

Heins, K. 1998. "Estrogen Q and A: Experts Answer Your Questions About the Female Hormone." *Better Homes and Gardens*, October, 144–46.

FINASTERIDE (PROPECIA)

American Academy of Dermatology. 1997. "New Treatment Options for Baldness Soon Available." ADA press release, March 23.

Editor. 1999. *Physicians' Desk Reference*. Montvale, N.J.: Medical Economics Company, Inc.

FLUTAMIDE (EULEXIN)

Editor. 1998. "Casodex/Bicalutamide." Internet website: www.regrowth.com.

Editor. 1999. *Physicians' Desk Reference*. Montvale, N.J.: Medical Economics Company, Inc.

IMMUNOSUPPRESSIVE DRUGS

Editor. 1999. *Physicians' Desk Reference*. Montvale, N.J.: Medical Economics Company, Inc.

Editor. 1993. *The PDR Family Guide to Prescription Drugs*. Montvale, N.J.: Medical Economics Data, Inc.

Gilhar, A., T. Pillar, and A. Etzioni. 1989. "Topical Cyclosporin A in Alopecia Areata." *Acta Dermato-Venereologica* 69: 252–53.

Mauduit, G., P. Lenvers, H. Barthelemy, and J. Thivolet. 1987. "Treatment of Severe Alopecia Areata with Topical Applications of Cyclosporin A." *Annales de Dermatologie et de Venereologie* 114: 507–10.

Oliver, R. F., and J. G. Lowe. 1995. "Oral Cyclosporin A Restores Hair Growth in the DEBR Rat Model for Alopecia Areata." *Clinical Experiments in Dermatology.* 20: 127–31.

Paquet, P., J. A. Estrada, and G. E. Pierard. 1992. "Oral Cyclosporin and Alopecia Areata." *Dermatology* 185: 314–15.

Shapiro, J., J. Tan, and V. Tron. 1997. "Systemic Cyclosporine and Low-Dose Prednisone in the Treatment of Chronic Severe Alopecia Areata: A Clinical and Immunopathologic Evaluation." *Journal of the American Academy of Dermatology* 36: 114–17.

Yamamoto, S., and R. Kato, 1994. "Hair Growth–Stimulating Effects of Cyclosporin A and FK506, Potent Immunosuppressants." *Journal of Dermatological Science* 7: S47–54.

ISOPRINOSINE

Galbraith, G.M., B. H. Thiers, J. Jensen, and F. Hoehler. 1987. "A Randomized Double-Blind Study of Inosiplex (Isoprinosine) Therapy in Patients with Alopecia Totalis." *Journal of the American Academy of Dermatology* 16 (5 pt 1): 977–83.

Life Extension Foundation. 1998. "Offshore Drugs." Internet website: www.
  lef.org.
PWA Health Group/The Body: An Aids and HIV Information Resource.
  1996. "Isoprinosine Info Sheet." Internet website: www.thebody.com/
  pwa/isop.html.
Thiers, B. H. 1991. "Isoprinosine Treatment of Alopecia Areata." *Journal of
  Investigative Dermatology* 96: 72S-73S.

KETOCONAZOLE (NIZORAL)
Editor. 1999. *Physicians' Desk Reference*. Montvale, N.J.: Medical Economics
  Company, Inc.
Editor. 1993. *The PDR Family Guide to Prescription Drugs*. Montvale, N.J.:
  Medical Economics Data, Inc.
Pierard-Franchimont, C., P. De Doncker, G. Cauwenbergh, and G. E. Pierard.
  1998. "Ketoconazole Shampoo: Effect of Long-Term Use in Androgenetic
  Alopecia." *Dermatology* 196: 474-77.

LIQUID NITROGEN
Editor. 1998. "Alopecia Areata." Internet website: www.follicle.com.

MINOXIDIL (ROGAINE)
Bamford, J. T. 1987. "A Falling Out Following Minoxidil: Telogen Effluvium."
  Journal of the American Academy of Dermatology 16 (1 pt 1): 144-46.
Bardelli, A., and A. Rebora. 1989. "Telogen Effluvium and Minoxidil." *Jour-
  nal of the American Academy of Dermatology* 21 (3 pt 1): 572-73.
Chriss, L. 1998. "Hair Loss: Facing the Fallout." *American Health for Women*,
  June, 22-24.
DeVillez, R. L., J. P. Jacobs, C. A. Szpunar, and M.L. Warner. 1994. "Androge-
  netic Alopecia in the Female. Treatment with 2% Topical Minoxidil Solu-
  tion." *Archives of Dermatology* 130: 303-307.
DeYarman Medical Group. 1998. "The Minoxidil Enhancement System."
  Internet website: www.deyarmanmedical.com.
Editor. 1999. *Physicians' Desk Reference*. Montvale, N.J.: Medical Economics
  Company, Inc.
Editor. 1993. *The PDR Family Guide to Prescription Drugs*. Montvale, N.J.:
  Medical Economics Data, Inc.
Editor. 1991. Rogaine for women. *The Doctor's People Newsletter*, October, 6.
Editor. 1998. "Treatment reviews." Internet web site: www.regrowth.com.
Fenton, D. A., and J. D. Wilkinson. 1983. "Topical Minoxidil in the Treatment
  of Alopecia Areata." *British Medical Journal* 8: 1015-17.
Folkenberg, J. 1988. "Hair Apparent? For Some, a New Solution to Baldness."
  FDA Consumer, December-January, 8-11.

Fransway, A. F., and S. A. Muller. 1988. "3 Percent Topical Minoxidil Compared with Placebo for the Treatment of Chronic Severe Alopecia Areata." *Cutis* 41: 431–35.

Frentz, G. 1985. "Topical Minoxidil for Extended Areata Alopecia." *Acta Dermato-Venereologica* 65: 172–75.

Granai, C. O., H. Frederickson, W. Gajewski, et al. 1991. "The Use of Minoxidil to Attempt to Prevent Alopecia During Chemotherapy for Gynecologic Malignancies." *European Journal of Gynaecological Oncology* 12: 129–32.

Hong, D., and L. L. Hart. 1990. "Topical Minoxidil for Women." *Annals of Pharmacotherapy* 24: 1062–63.

Jacobs, J. P., C. A. Szpunar, and M. L. Warner. 1993. "Use of Topical Minoxidil Therapy for Androgenetic Alopecia in Women." *International Journal of Dermatology* 32: 758–62.

Olsen, E. A. 1991. "Topical Minoxidil in the Treatment of Androgenetic Alopecia in Women." *Cutis* 48: 243–48.

Patton, S. 1998. *The Facts About Hair Regrowth.* Kalamazoo, Mich.: Pharmacia & Upjohn.

Price, V. H. 1987. "Double-Blind, Placebo-Controlled Evaluation of Topical Minoxidil in Extensive Alopecia Areata." *Journal of the American Academy of Dermatology* 16 (3 pt 2): 730–36.

Price, V. H., and E. Menefee. 1990. "Quantitative Estimation of Hair Growth. Androgenetic Alopecia in Women: Effect of Minoxidil." *Journal of Investigative Dermatology* 95: 683–87.

Ranchoff, R. E., W. F. Bergfeld, W. D. Steck, and S. J. Subichin. 1989. "Extensive Alopecia Areata. Results of Treatment with 3% Topical Minoxidil." *Cleveland Clinic Journal of Medicine* 56: 149–54.

Shapiro, J., and V. Price. 1998. "Hair Regrowth—Therapeutic Agents." *Dermatologic Clinics* 16: 341–56.

Whiting, D. A., and C. Jacobsen. "Treatment of Female Androgenetic Alopecia with Minoxidil 2%." *International Journal of Dermatology* 31: 800–804.

Tse, D. 1997. *Hair Loss Treatment Almanac 1998.* New York: TSE Publishing, Inc.

PROXIPHEN

Editor. 1998a. "Proxiphen." Internet website: www.regrowth.com.

Editor. 1998b. "Proxiphen." Internet website: www.drproctor.com.

PUVA (PSORALENS AND ULTRAVIOLET LIGHT)

Amer, M. A., and A. El Garf. 1983. "Photochemotherapy and Alopecia Areata." *International Journal of Dermatology* 22: 245–46.

Claudy, A. L., and D. Gagnaire. 1983. "PUVA Treatment of Alopecia Areata." *Archives of Dermatology* 119: 975–78.

Healy, E., and S. Rogers. 1993. "PUVA Treatment for Alopecia Areata—Does It Work? A Retrospective Review of 102 Cases." *British Journal of Dermatology* 129: 42–44.

Lassus A., U. Kianto, E. Johansson, and T. Juvakoski. 1980. "PUVA Treatment for Alopecia Areata." *Dermatologica* 161: 298–304.

———. 1984. "Treatment of Alopecia Areata with Three Different PUVA Modalities." *Photodermatology* 1: 141–44.

Sahin S., B. Yalcin, and A. Karaduman. 1998. "PUVA Treatment for Alopecia Areata. Experience in a Turkish Population." *Dermatology* 197: 245–47.

Van der Schaar, W. W., and J. H. Sillevis Smith. 1984. "An Evaluation of PUVA-Therapy for Alopecia Areata." *Dermatologica* 168: 250–52.

SPIRONOLACTONE (ALDACTONE)

Akamatsu, H., C. C. Zouboulis, and C. E. Orfanos. 1993. "Spironolactone Directly Inhibits Proliferation of Cultured Human Facial Sebocytes and Acts Antagonistically to Testosterone and 5 Alpha-Dihydrotestosterone in Vitro." *Journal of Investigative Dermatology* 100: 660–62.

Blanchard, G., and B. Blanchard. 1989. "Approach to Hair Loss Reduction." *Journal of the National Medical Association* 81: 755–56.

Callan, A. W., and J. Montalto. 1995. "Female Androgenetic Alopecia: An Update." *Australasian Journal of Dermatology* 36: 51–55.

Diamanti-Kandarakis, E., G. Tolis, and A. J. Duleba. 1995. "Androgens and Therapeutic Aspects of Antiandrogens in Women." *Journal of the Society for Gynecologic Investigation* 2: 577–92.

Editor. 1999. *Physicians' Desk Reference.* Montvale, N.J.: Medical Economics Company, Inc.

Editor. 1993. *The PDR Family Guide to Prescription Drugs.* Montvale, N.J.: Medical Economics Data, Inc.

THYMOPENTIN

Orecchia, G. 1989. "Thymopentin in the Treatment of Alopecia Areata." *Dermatologica* 178: 231.

TOPICAL CONTACT SENSITIZATION THERAPY

Berth-Jones, J., and P. E. Hutchinson. 1991. "Treatment of Alopecia Totalis with a Combination of Inosine Pranobex and Diphencyprone Compared to Each Treatment Alone." *Clinical Experiments in Dermatology* 16: 172–75.

Case, P. C., J. A. Mitchell, N. A. Swanson, et al. 1984. "Topical Therapy of Alopecia Areata with Squaric Acid Dibutylester." *Journal of the American Academy of Dermatology* 10: 447–50.

Caserio, R. J. 1987. "Treatment of Alopecia Areata with Squaric Acid Dibutylester." *Archives of Dermatology* 123: 1036–41.

Chiarappa, M., and L. Harris. 1996. "I Went Bald at 33." *Ladies Home Journal*, June, 36–38.

Chua, S. H., C. L. Goh, and C. B. Ang. 1996. "Topical Squaric Acid Dibutylester Therapy for Alopecia Areata: A Double-Sided Patient Controlled Study." *Annals of the Academy of Medicine of Singapore* 25: 842–47.

Daman, L. A., E. W. Rosenberg, and L. Drake. 1978. "Treatment of Alopecia Areata with Dinitrochlorobenzene." *Archives of Dermatology* 114: 1036–38.

De Prost, Y., F. R. Paquez, and R. Touraine. 1979. "Treatment of Alopecia Areata with DNCB." *Annales de Dermatologie et de Venereologie*106: 437–40.

———. 1982. "Dinitrochlorobenzene Treatment of Alopecia Areata." *Archives of Dermatology* 118: 542–45.

Frentz, G., and K. Eriksen. 1977. "Treatment of Alopecia Areata with DNCB—an Immunostimulation?" *Acta Dermato-Venereologica* 57: 370–71.

Friedmann, P. S. 1981. "Response of Alopecia Areata to DNCB: Influence of Auto-Antibodies and Route of Sensitization." *British Journal of Dermatology* 105: 285–89.

Gutschmidt, E. 1979. "Contribution to the DNCB Therapy of Alopecia Areata." *Zeitschrift für Hautkrankheiten* 54: 430–35.

Happle, R. 1979. "DNCB Therapy of Alopecia Areata." *Zeitschrift für Hautkrankheiten* 54: 426–29.

Happle, R., K. Cebulla, and K. Echternacht-Happle. 1978. "Dinitrochlorobenzene Therapy for Alopecia Areata." *Archives of Dermatology* 114: 1629–31.

Happle, R., and K. Echternacht. 1977. "Induction of Hair Growth in Alopecia Areata with DNCB." *Lancet* 12: 1002–1003.

Happle, R., B. M. Hausen, and L. Wiesner-Menzel. 1983. "Diphencyprone in the Treatment of Alopecia Areata." *Acta Dermato-Venereologica* 63: 49–52.

Happle, R., K. J. Kalveram, U. Buchner, et al. "Contact Allergy as a Therapeutic Tool for Alopecia Areata: Application of Squaric Acid Dibutylester." *Dermatologica* 161: 289–97.

Hoting, E., and A. Boehm. 1992. "Therapy of Alopecia Areata with Diphencyprone." *British Journal of Dermatology* 127: 625–29.

Johansson, E., A. Ranki, T. Reunala, et al. "Immunohistological Evaluation of Alopecia Areata Treated with Squaric Acid Dibutylester (SADBE)." *Acta Dermato-Venereologica* 66: 485–90.

Kalam, A., M. D. Tahseen, S. F. Islam, et al. "Dinitrochlorobenzene Therapy in Alopecia Areata." *Journal of the Indiana Medical Association* 89: 9–10.

Kietzmann, H., H. Hardung, and E. Christophers. 1985. "Therapy of Alopecia Areata with Diphenylcyclopropenone." *Hautarzt* 36: 331–35.

Lindemayr, H. 1981. "Disappointing Results with Dinitrochlorobenzene in Alopecia Areata." *Wiener Klinische Wochenschrift* 93: 131–34.

Micali, G., R. L. Cicero, M. R. Nasca, and A. Sapuppo, 1996. "Treatment of Alopecia Areata with Squaric Acid Dibutylester." *International Journal of Dermatology* 35: 52–56.

Ochsendorf, F. R., G. Mitrou, and R. Milbradt. 1988. "Therapy of Alopecia Areata with Diphenylcyclopropenone." *Zeitschrift für Hautkrankheiten* 63: 94, 96, 99–100.

Shapiro, J. 1993. "Topical Immunotherapy in the Treatment of Chronic Severe Alopecia Areata." *Dermatologic Clinics* 11: 611–17.

Shapiro, J., J. Tan, V. Ho, and F. Abbott. 1993. "Treatment of Chronic Severe Alopecia Areata with Topical Diphenylcyclopropenone and 5% Minoxidil: A Clinical and Immunopathologic Evaluation." *Journal of the American Academy of Dermatology* 29: (5 pt 1): 729–35.

Temmerman, L., J. de Weert, L. de Keyser, and A. Lint. 1984. "Treatment of Alopecia Areata with Dinitrochlorobenzene." *Acta Dermato-Venereologica* 64: 441–43.

Valsecchi, R., T. Cainelli, L. Foiadelli, and A. Rossi. 1986. "Topical Immunotherapy of Alopecia Areata. A Follow-Up Study." *Acta Dermato-Venereologica* 66: 269–72.

Van der Steen, P. H., H. M. Van Baar, C. M. Perret, and R. Happle. 1991. "Treatment of Alopecia Areata with Diphenylcyclopropenone." *Journal of the American Academy of Dermatology* 24 (2 pt 1): 253–57.

TRETINOIN (RETIN-A)

Bazzano, G. S., N. Terezakis, and W. Galen. 1986. "Topical Tretinoin for Hair Growth." *Journal of the American Academy of Dermatology* 15: 880–83, 890–93.

Bazzano, G. S., N. Terezakis, H. Attia, et al. 1993. "Effect of Retinoids on Follicular Cells." *Journal of Investigative Dermatology* 101: 138S–142S.

Bergfeld, W. F. 1998. "Retinoids and Hair Growth." *Journal of the American Academy of Dermatology* 39: S86–S89.

Editor. 1990. "Aspects of Retinoids." *American Family Physician* 41: 950.

Editor. 1998a. "Medical Study Finds Combination Formula Most Effective for Regrowing Women's Hair." *National Women's Review*, Summer-Fall, 1.

Editor. 1997. "New Medical Study Shows Combination Formula More Effective in Regrowing Hair." *Atlanta Sports and Fitness Magazine*, February.

Editor. 1998b. "Replacing Lost Hair." *New York Post*, April 6.

Editor. 1999. *Physicians' Desk Reference*. Montvale, N.J.: Medical Economics Company, Inc.

Editor. 1993. *The PDR Family Guide to Prescription Drugs*. Montvale, N.J.: Medical Economics Data, Inc.

Editor. 1998c. "Retin-A/Tretinoin." Internet website: www.regrowth.com.

Lewenberg, A. "Dr. Lewenberg's Formula." Promotional material.

Tse, D. 1997. *Hair Loss Treatment Almanac 1998*. New York: TSE Publishing, Inc.

XANDROX

Editor. 1998. "Xandrox." Internet website: www.minoxidil.com.

Chapter Five

Christian, J. S. 1994. "A Review of the Pharmacology, Clinical Applications, and Toxicology of Thymopentin." *Transgenica—The Journal of Clinical Biotechnology* 1; 23–34.

Editor. 1999a. "Aminexil: A Major Scientific Discovery in Preventing Hair Loss." Internet website: www.loreal.com.

Editor. 1988a. "A 'Magic Liquid' for Hair?" *Newsweek*, March 28, available at Internet website: www.fabao.com.

Editor. 1998b. "Dercap/Aminexil." Internet website: www.regrowth.com.

Editor. 1998c. "Fabao 101D." Internet website: www.fabao.com.

Editor. 1998d. "Folligen/copper peptone." Internet website: www.regrowth.com.

Editor. 1999b. "Folligen." Internet website: www.skinbio.com.

Editor. 1999c. "Kevis." Internet website: www.kevisnet.

Editor. 1998e. "Nioxin." Internet website: www.nioxin.com.

Editor. 1998f. "Rhodanide Replenisher Facts." Internet website: www.rhodanide.com

Editor. 1998g. "Thymu-Skin Works." Internet website: www.microhosting.com/alopecia/.

Editor. 1998h. "Tricomin." Internet website: www.tricomin.com.

Gargan, E. A. 1988. "In Baldness War, Rumors of Advance for Hairline." *New York Times*, January 26, available at Internet website: www.fabao.com.

Gruber, D. M., M. O. Sator, E. M. Kokoschka, and J. C. Huber. 1998. "Thymopentin in Alopecia Areata." *Acta Medica Austriaca* 25: 33–35.

Hanover, L. 1997. "Hair Replacement: What Works, What Doesn't." *FDA Consumer*, April, 7–11.

Kessels, A. G. H., R. L. L. M. Cardynaals, R. L. L. Borger, et al. 1991. "The

Effectiveness of the Hair Restorer 'Fabao' in Males with Alopecia Andro-genetica. A Clinical Experiment." *Journal of Clinical Epidemiology* 44: 439–47.

Kramer, A., W. Weuffen, S. Minnich, et al. 1990. "Promotion of Hair Growth with Thiocyanate in Guinea Pigs." *Dermatologische Monatsschrift* 176: 417–20.

Lee, K. S., K. B. Myung, and H. I. Kook. 1987. "A Clinical Study of Topical Mucopolysaccharides and Polydeoxyribonucleoprotein (Foltene) Ther-apy in Alopecia." *Journal of Korean Medical Science* 2: 157–65.

Mahé, Y. F., B. Buan, and B. A. Bernard. 1996. "A Minoxidil-Related Com-pound Lacking a C6 Substitution Still Exhibits Strong Anti-Lysyl Hydroxylase Activity in Vitro." *Skin Pharmacology* 9: 177–83.

NISIM New Hair Biofactors. Promotional materials.

Qian, B. C., J. Chen, and H. J. Xu. 1994. "Pharmacological Action of 101-B Hair Regeneration Extract on Skin and Hair in Experimental Animals." *Chung Kuo Chung His I Chieh Ho Tsa Chih* 14: 227–29.

Raztec, N. "Crinagen." Internet website: www.raztec.com.

Tosti, A., P. Manuzzi, and A. Gasponi. 1988. "Thymopentin in the Treatment of Severe Alopecia Areata." *Dermatologica* 177: 170–74.

Tse, D. 1997. *Hair Loss Treatment Almanac 1998.* New York: TSE Publishing, Inc.

Weuffen, W., A. Kramer, B. Thurkow, and H. Winetzka. 1994. "Effect of an Alimentary Thiocyanate Supplement on the Hide Characteristics of Mink." *Berliner Und Munchener Tierarztliche Wochenschrift* 107: 299–302.

Chapter Six

Bergfeld, W. F. 1978. "Diffuse Hair Loss in Women." *Cutis* 22: 190–95.

Editor. 1997. "Hair You Love—How to Have It Now." *Good Housekeeping,* February, 40–42.

Editor. 1998. "Hairy Conniption." *Cosmopolitan,* February, 264–66.

Editor. 1994. "How To (Finally!) Love Your Hair." *Redbook,* August, 90–95.

Editor. 1995. "Top Condition." *Redbook,* February, 100–103.

Liberty, M. 1994. "Fresh Hair Care Routine." *Better Nutrition,* October, 64–67.

Rushton, D. H., P. Kingsley, and N. L. Neil. 1993. "Treating Reduced Hair Volume in Women." *Cosmetics and Toiletries* 108: 59–62.

Sharp, K. 1996. "What to Do About Bad Hair Days." *Current Health* 2, March, 16–18.

Chapter Seven

Current Technology Corporation. 1998. "Corporate Overview and ETG Technology." Internet website: www.currentech.com.

Fayerman, P. 1997. "A Hair-Raising Story." *Vancouver Sun*, July 21.

Judd, N. 1996. "Plugging into a Growth Industry." *Vancouver Courier*, September 8.

Kornhauser, S. H., and W. S. Maddin. 1992. "ETG—Electrotrichogenesis." *American Journal of Electromedicine*. Available at Internet website: www.currentech.com.

Maddin, W. S., and I. Amara, and W. A. Sollecito. 1992. "Electrotrichogenesis: Further Evidence of Efficacy and Safety of Extended Use." *International Journal of Dermatology* 31: 878–80.

Maddin, W. S., P. W. Bell, and J. H. M. James. 1990. "The Biological Effects of a Pulsed Electrostatic Field with Specific Reference to Hair." *International Journal of Dermatology* 29: 446–50.

Chapter Eight

Hughes, L. 1996. "Beauty in a Pill: Are Supplements Today's Fountain of Youth?" *Environmental Nutrition*, May, 1-2.

Liberty, M. 1993. "Healthier Hair." *Better Nutrition*, May, 56–59.

Chapter Nine

Berdanier, C. D. 1992. "Is Inositol an Essential Nutrient?" *Nutrition Today* 27: 22–26.

Crayhorn, R. J. 1996. "Vitamins: The Basics." *Total Health*, April, 26–28.

Colombo, V. E., F. Gerber, M. Bronhofer, and G. L. Floersheim, 1990. "Treatment of Brittle Fingernails and Onychoschizia with Biotin: Scanning Electron Microscopy." *Journal of the American Academy of Dermatology* 23: 1127–32.

Editor. 1999. "Natural Vitamin E Superior to Synthetic." *Nutritional Outlook*, January-February, 56.

Kirschmann, J. D. 1979. *Nutrition Almanac*. New York: McGraw-Hill Book Company.

Kniewald, Z., V. Zechner, and J. Kniewald. 1992. "Androgen Hydroxysteroid Dehydrogenases Under the Influence of Pyridoxine Derivatives." *Endocrine Regulations* 26: 47–51.

Kurtzweil, P. 1991. "Biotin." *FDA Consumer*, October, 34.

Lombard, K. A., and D. M. Mock. 1989. "Biotin Nutritional Status of Vegans, Lactoovovegetarians, and Nonvegetarians." *American Journal of Clinical Nutrition* 50: 486–90.

Mestel, R. 1998. "Beautiful Skin from A to E." *Health*, October, 72–75.

Pawlowski, A., and W. Kostanecki. 1966. "Effect of Biotin on Hair Roots and Sebum Excretion in Women with Diffuse Alopecia." *Polish Medical Journal* 5: 447–52.

Peters, K., D. Stuss, and N. Waddell. 1994. *Hair Loss Prevention Through Natural Remedies: A Prescription for Healthier Hair*. Vancouver, British Columbia: Apple Publishing Company, Ltd.

Chapter Ten

Ead, R. D. 1981. "Oral Zinc Sulphate in Alopecia Areata—a Double Blind Trial." *British Journal of Dermatology* 104: 483.

Editor. 1995. "Silica Is Crucial for Nails, Hair and Bones." *Better Nutrition*, December, 30.

Hunt, C. D., T. R. Shuler, and L. M. Mullen. 1991. "Concentration of Boron and Other Elements in Human Foods and Personal-Care Products." *Journal of the American Dietetic Association* 91: 558–68.

Johnson, M. A., and S. E. Kays. 1990. "Copper: Its Role in Human Nutrition." *Nutrition Today*, February, 6–14.

Kirschmann, J. D. 1979. *Nutrition Almanac*. New York: McGraw-Hill Book Company.

Mitchell, J. 1991. "Many Riches to Be Mined from Minerals." *Health News & Review*, December, 6.

Murray, F. 1989. "Copper Essential for Healthy Skin and Hair." *Better Nutrition*, February, 18–19.

———. 1990. "Zinc: A Vital Skin and Hair Mineral." *Better Nutrition*, July, 12–14.

Peters, K., D. Stuss, and N. Waddell. 1994. *Hair Loss Prevention Through Natural Remedies: A Prescription for Healthier Hair*. Vancouver, British Columbia: Apple Publishing Company, Ltd.

Chapter Eleven

Balch, J. F., and P. A. Balch. 1997. *Prescription for Nutritional Healing*. 2nd ed. New York: Avery Publishing Company.

Hertel, H., H. Gollnick, C. Matties, et al. 1989. "Low Dosage Retinol and L-Cystine Combination Improve Alopecia of the Diffuse Type Following Long-Term Oral Administration." *Hautarzt* 40: 490–95.

Chapter Twelve

Aruoma, O. I., B. Halliwell, R. Aeschbach, and J. Loligers. 1992. "Antioxidant and Pro-Oxidant Properties of Active Rosemary Constituents: Carnosol and Carnosic Acid." *Xenobiotica* 22: 257–68.

Balch, J. F., and P. A. Balch. 1997. *Prescription for Nutritional Healing.* 2nd ed. New York: Avery Publishing Company.

Blumenthal, M. 1998. *The Complete German Commission E Monographs: Therapeutic Guide to Herbal Medicines.* Austin, Tex: American Botanical Council.

Brown, D. 1990. "The Male Dilemma: Relief for Prostate Problems." *Total Health*, June, 40–41.

But, P. P., B. Tomlinson, and K. L. Lee. 1996. "Hepatitis Related to the Chinese Medicine Shou-Wu-Pian Manufactured from Polygonum Multiflorum." *Veterinary and Human Toxicology* 38: 280–82.

Dolby, V. 1997. "Asian Anti-Aging Secrets: Green Tea and Soy." *Better Nutrition*, February, 22–24.

Foster, S. 1997. "Kava-Kava, a Gift of Calm from the South Pacific." *Better Nutrition*, May, 54–58.

Gormley, J. J. 1996. "For Wound Healing, Silicon-Rich Horsetail Makes Good 'Horse Sense.'" *Better Nutrition*, May, 30.

Editor. 1998a. "Alopecia Info & Resources: Green Tea." Internet website: www.follicle.com.

Editor. 1998b. "Green Tea Ingredient Kills Cancer Cells, Spares Healthy Ones." *Cancer Weekly Plus*, January 5, 5.

Editor. 1998c. "Tegreen: A Cup of Tea in a Pill?" *Environmental Nutrition* 21: 3.

Hobbs, C. 1991. "Adaptogens: All-Purpose Herbs." *East West*, July-August, 54–61.

Hryb, D. J., M. S. Khan, N. A. Romas, and W. Rosner. 1995. "The Effect of Extracts of the Roots of the Stinging Nettle (Urtica Dioica) on the Interaction of SHBG with Its Receptor on Human Prostatic Membranes." *Planta Medica* 61: 31–32.

Hunter, Beatrice Trum. 1995. "An Unsafe Medicinal Tea?" *Consumers' Research Magazine*, August, 8-9.

Inaoka, Y., A. Shakuya, H. Fukazawa, et al. 1994. "Studies on Active Substances in Herbs Used for Hair Treatment. Effects of Herb Extracts on Hair Growth and Isolation of an Active Substance from Polyporus Umbellatus F." *Chemical and Pharmaceutical Bulletin* 42: 530–33.

Kim, S. H., K. S. Jeong, S. Y. Ryu, and T. H. Kim. 1998. "Panax Ginseng Prevents Apoptosis in Hair Follicles and Accelerates Recovery of Hair Medullary Cells in Irradiated Mice." *In Vivo* 12: 219–22.

Kobayashi, N., R. Suzuki, C. Koide, et al. 1993. "Effect of Leaves of Gingko Biloba on Hair Regrowth in C3H Strain Mice." *Yakugaku Zasshi* 113: 718–24.

Kobren, S. D. 1998. "The Bald Truth." New York: Pocket Books.

Liao, S., and R. A. Hiipaka. 1995. "Selective Inhibition of Steroid 5 Alpha-Reductase Isozymes by Tea Epicatechin-3-Gallate and Epigallocatechin-3-Gallate." *Biochemical and Biophysical Research Communications* 214: 833–38.

Liberati, M. 1996. "Mother Nature Knows Best for Shampoos and Conditioners. *Better Nutrition*, March, 76–78.

Liberty, M. 1993. "Healthier Hair." *Better Nutrition*, May, 56–59.

Miles, K. 1992. "Natural Hair Care." *Mothering*, Summer, 58–63.

O'Connor, A. 1997. "Getting to the Root of Beautiful Hair: Shiny, Silky Hair Begins with a Healthy Scalp." *Vegetarian Times*, October, 112–14.

O'Donnell, S. A. 1999. "Herbs to Replace Wigs?" *Prevention*, May, 49.

Peters, K., D. Stuss, and N. Waddell. 1994. *Hair Loss Prevention Through Natural Remedies: A Prescription for Healthier Hair.* Vancouver, British Columbia: Apple Publishing Company, Ltd.

Schindler, M. 1996. "Natural Beauty Solutions: Want Smooth Skin, a Radiant Complexion, and Healthy Hair? It's Easy with These 25 Simple and Effective Home Remedies." *Natural Health*, March-April, 92–99.

Skolnick, P., W. H. Eagelstein, and V. A. Ziboh. 1977. "Human Essential Fatty Acid Deficiency: Treatment by Topical Application of Linoleic Acid." *Archives of Dermatology* 113: 939–41.

Steinman, D. 1994. "Enlarged Prostate? Try Tree Bark." *Natural Health*, July-August, 44–46.

Sultan, C., A. Terraza, C. Devillier, et al. 1984. "Inhibition of Androgen Metabolism and Binding by a Liposterolic Extract of 'Serona Repens B' in Human Foreskin Fibroblasts." *Journal of Steroid Biochemistry* 20: 515–19.

Tse, D. 1997. *Hair Loss Treatment Almanac 1998.* New York: TSE Publishing, Inc.

Tyler, V. E. 1994. "Questionable Herbal Products." *Nutrition Forum.* November-December, 53–56.

———. 1997. "Nature's Stress Buster." *Prevention*, October, 90–93.

Walji, H. 1997. *Kava: Nature's Relaxant.* Prescott, Ariz.: Hohm Press.

York, J., T. Nicholson, P. Minors, and D. F. Duncan. 1998. "Stressful Life

Events and Loss of Hair Among Adult Women, a Case-Controlled Study."
Psychological Reports 82 (3 pt 1): 1044–46.

Zalka, A. D., J. A. Byarlay, and L. A. Goldsmith. 1994. "Alopecia à Deux: Simultaneous Occurrence of Alopecia in a Husband and Wife." *Archives of Dermatology* 130: 390–92.

Chapter Thirteen

Adams, R., and F. Murray. 1979. *Health Foods*. New York: Larchmont Books.

Kirschmann, J. D. 1979. *Nutrition Almanac*. New York: McGraw-Hill Book Company.

Lassus, A., and E. Eskelinen. 1992. "A Comparative Study of a New Food Supplement, Viviscal, with Fish Extract for the Treatment of Hereditary Androgenetic Alopecia in Young Males." *Journal of International Medical Research* 20: 445–53.

Lower, E. 1996. "Royal Jelly Gives a Buzz to Skin Care Formulations." *Manufacturing Chemist* 67: 41.

Mindell, E. 1996. *What You Should Know About Beautiful Hair, Skin and Nails*. New Canaan, Conn.: Keats Publishing, Inc.

———. 1998. *Earl Mindell's Supplement Bible*. New York: Fireside.

Murray, F. 1991. "Get the Buzz on Bee Pollen." *Better Nutrition*, May, 20–22.

Orr, T. B. 1998. "Royal Jelly from the Beehive: Fit for a Queen." *Better Nutrition*, July, 34.

Scheer, J. F. 1993. "Royal Jelly: Health and Life Enhancer." *Better Nutrition*, December, 30–34.

Chapter Fourteen

American Hair Loss Council. 1998. "What Is Hair Replacement Surgery?" Internet website: www.ahlc.org.

American Society of Plastic and Recontructive Surgeons. 1993. "Hair Replacement Surgery." Internet website: www.plasticsurgery.org.

Barrera, A. 1997. "Micrograft and Minigraft Megasession Hair Transplantation Results After a Single Session." *Plastic and Reconstructive Surgery* 100: 1524–30.

Bernstein, R. M. 1996. "Hair Restoration: Answered Questions." *Dermatologic Surgery* 22: 95–98.

Bernstein, R. M., and W. R. Rassman. 1997. "Follicular Transplantation—Patient Evaluation and Surgical Planning." *Dermatologic Surgery* 23; 771–84.

————. 1996. "Laser Hair Transplantation: Is It Really State of the Art?" *Lasers in Surgery and Medicine* 19: 233–35.

————. 1998a. "Rapid Fire Hair Implanter Carousel." *Dermatologic Surgery* 24: 623–27.

————. 1998b. "Standardizing the Classification and Description of Follicular Unit Transplantation and Mini- And Micrografting Techniques." *Dermatologic Surgery* 24: 957–63.

Bertucci, V., D. Berg, and S. V. Pollack. 1998. "Hair Transplantation Update." *Journal of Cutaneous Medicine and Surgery* 2: 180–86.

Burke, K. E. 1989. "Hair Loss: What Causes It and What Can Be Done About It." *Postgraduate Medicine* 85: 52–77.

Camps-Fresneda, A. 1994. "Age and Patient Selection in Planning Hair Transplantation Procedures." *Journal of Dermatologic Surgery and Oncology* 20: 221.

Cotterill, P. C., and W. P. Unger. 1992. "Hair Transplantation in Females." *Journal of Dermatologic Surgery and Oncology* 18: 477–81.

Earles, R. M. 1986. "Surgical Correction of Traumatic Alopecia Marginalis or Traction Alopecia in Black Women." *Journal of Dermatologic Surgery and Oncology* 12: 78–82.

Editor. 1988. "Hair-Raising Possibilities: Coping in an Age of Creeping Baldness." *Total Health*, June, 14–16.

Editor. 1994. "The Latest on Baldness Cures." *Health News*, December, 4-6.

Farber, G. A. 1982. "The Punch Scalp Graft." *Clinics in Plastic Surgery* 9: 207–20.

Griffin, E. I. 1995. "Hair Transplantation: The Fourth Decade." *Dermatologic Clinics* 13: 363–87.

Halsner, U. E., and M. W. G. Lucas. 1995. "New Aspects in Hair Transplantation for Females." *Dermatologic Surgery* 21: 605–10.

Hanke, C. W. 1981. "Hair Implants vs. Hair Transplants." *Journal of the American Medical Association* 246: 1405.

Kobren, S. D. 1998. *The Bald Truth*. New York: Pocket Books.

Norwood, O. T. 1992. "Patient Selection, Hair Transplant Design, and Hairstyle." *Journal of Dermatologic Surgery and Oncology* 18: 386–94.

Norwood Lehr Hair Transplant Clinic. 1998. "Follicular Transplantation." Internet website: www.hairclinic.com.

Orbay, A. S., and O. A. Dysal. 1998. "A New Dilator for Hair Transplantation." *Plastic and Recontructive Surgery* 101: 222–24.

Pinski, J. B., and K. S. Pinski. 1987. "New Aspects of Hair Transplantation." *Cutis* 309–13.

Riggs, P. 1998. "Laser Hair Transplantation." Internet website: www. regrowth.com.

Smith, J. 1996. "Gone Today, Hair Tomorrow." *Town and Country Monthly*, April, 110–14.

Stough, D., F. Jimenez, and M. Avram. 1995. "Hair: Don't Stop Thinking About Tomorrow—It'll Soon Be Here." *Dermatologic Surgery* 21: 415–16.

Stough, D. B., B. J. Schell, and R. P. Weyrich. 1997. "The Role of Facial Proportion in Hair Restoration Surgery." *Annals of Plastic Surgery* 38: 129–36.

Swinehart, J. M., and E. I. Griffin. 1991. "Slit Grafting: The Use of Serrated Island Grafts in Male and Female-Pattern Alopecia." *Journal of Dermatologic Surgery and Oncology* 17: 243–53.

Chapter Fifteen

American Hair Loss Council. 1998. "What Is a Non-Surgical Hair Addition?" Internet website: www.ahlc.com.

Editor. 1998a. "Folligraft." Internet website: www.folligraft.com.

Editor. 1998b. "Regrowth" Internet website: www.regrowth.com.

Editor. 1999a. "Transdermal Hair Restoration." Internet website: www.emerging-solutions.com.

Editor. 1999b. "United Micro Systems, Inc." Internet website: www.unitedmicrosystems.com.

Gaudoin, T. 1992. "Wig It." *Harper's Bazaar*, November, 132–34.

Hanover, L. 1997. "Hair Replacement: What Works, What Doesn't." *FDA Consumer*, April, 7–11.

Weinstock, C. P. 1998. "Cosmetic Help for Cancer Patients." Internet website: www.fda.gov.

Epilogue

Editor. 1998a. "Antiandrogens." Internet website: www.regrowth.com.

Editor. 1998b. "Culturing Hair Matrix Cells to Produce Unlimited Amounts of Donor Hair." Internet website: www.regrowth.com.

Editor. 1998c. "Estrogen Blocker Grows Hair." Internet website: www.regrowth.com.

Editor. 1998d. "Gene Therapy." Internet website: www.regrowth.com.

Editor. 1998e. "Gene May Hold Cure to Baldness." Internet website: www.regrowth.com.

Editor. 1998f. "Interview with Michael Holick." Internet website: www.regrowth.com.

Henahan, S. 1998. "Gene Juice for Falling Follicles?" Internet website: www.regrowth.com.

Holick, M. F., S. Ray, T. C. Chen, et al. 1994. "A Parathyroid Hormone Antagonist Stimulates Epidermal Proliferation and Hair Growth in Mice." *Proceedings of the National Academy of Science* 91: 8014–16.

Kobren, S. D. 1998. *The Bald Truth*. New York: Pocket Books.

Oh, H. S., and R. C. Smart. 1996. "An Estrogen Receptor Pathway Regulates the Telogen-Anagen Hair Follicle Transition and Influences Epidermal Cell Proliferation." *Proceedings of the National Academy of Sciences* 93: 12525–30.

Senior, K. 1998. "B-Catenin Identified as Epithelial Signal That Induces Hair Morphogenesis." *Lancet* 352: 1761.

Uno, H., J. W. Kemnitz, and A. Cappas. 1990. "The Effects of Topical Diazoxide on Hair Follicular Growth and Physiology of the Stumptailed Macaque." *Journal of Dermatological Science* 1: 183–94.

Appendix C

Associated Press. 1998. "*WWW.Consumers* Buying Drugs." *The Evansville* (Indiana) *Courier*, December 22, A-15.

Index

Disease, 32–34, 39, 67, 186, 190.
    See also specific disease or condition
DMG (dimethylglycine), 178–79
DNCB (dinitorchlorobenzene), 77–79
Donor hair, 212–13, 214
DPCP (diphenylcyclopropene), 77–79
Drithocreme/Drithro-Scalp. *See*
    Anthralin
Drugs
    as cause of hair loss, 29, 31, 39, 67
    purchasing, 229–32
    See also specific category of drugs or
        drug
Dyes/bleaches, 35, 98

ElectroTrichoGenesis (ETG), 20,
    121–23
Essential fatty acid supplements (EFAs),
    179–80
Estrogen, 17, 19, 29, 53, 54–56, 144,
    212, 213
Ethnicity, 10
Eulexin, 57–59
Eumelanin, 10
Eyebrow/eyelash hair, 28, 71

Fabao 101, 94–97
Female-pattern baldness, 15. *See also*
    Androgenetic alopecia
Ferritin, 41, 149–50, 154
Fibrosis, 90, 196
Finasteride, 45, 56–57, 67, 89, 211
5 alpha reductase, 15, 179
    and androgenetic alopecia, 19, 93
    and DHT-testosterone conversion, 15,
        19, 46–47, 55, 56, 93, 131
    and future hair savers, 211–12
    and herbs, 163, 167, 168
Flap surgery, 199
Fluocinolone acetonide, 50
Flutamide (Eulexin), 57–59
Fo-ti (ho shou wu), 161–62
Follicles
    electrical stimulation of, 123
    and hair growth, 8–10, 12
    and types of hair, 11
    See also DHT-testerone conversion;
        specific condition or treatment

Follicular unit transplantation, 193–94,
    197
Folliculitis, 33, 196
Folligen, 97–99
Folligraft, 208
Foltene, 99–101
Food and Drug Administration, U.S.
    (FDA)
    and antiandrogens, 18
    and grafts/transplants, 190, 198, 208
    and hair relaxers, 35
    and nondrug treatments, 89
    and nutritional supplements, 182
    Thymu-Skin approval by, 110
    See also specific drug
Fungal infections, 33, 34, 39

Gene therapy, 213–14
Genetics, 26, 29, 39. *See also*
    Androgenetic alopecia
Ginger, 95
Ginkgo, 92, 93, 163
Ginseng, 95, 108, 162–63
Grafts, hair, 190, 191–94, 196–98, 199,
    200, 201, 207
Green tea, 163–64
Griffin, Edmond, 188

Hair
    functions of, 7
    growth of, 8–10, 11–13
    psychological effects of, 3, 7, 154
    self-education about, 4
    types of human, 10–11
Hair care products, 173–74, 229–32. *See*
    also Conditioners; Shampoos
Hair loss
    causes of, 38–41, 95
    diagnosis of, 38–41, 85, 154
    in future, 211–15
    statistics about, 3, 24
    See also specific condition or treatment
Hair relaxers, 35
Hair shafts, 19, 116
Hair systems, 202, 207–9
Hair transplants, 4, 5, 20, 98, 185–98,
    208–9, 214
Hair weaving, 202

finasteride compared with, 56
and how it is used, 68–69
and how it works, 63–64, 72
length of time for results with,
70–71
as over-the-counter drug, 37, 45, 63
as prescription drug, 45, 63
in shampoos, 113
side effects of, 65, 71
and surgery, 197
and telogen effluvium, 66–67
Minoxidil-like medicines, 214
MK-386, 211
MK-0434, 211
MK-0963, 211

National Alopecia Areata Foundation
(NAAF), 27, 223
National Institutes of Health (NIH), 6
Niacin, 93, 108, 141, 142
Nioxin, 23, 108–9
Nisim New Hair Biofactors, 23, 103–5
Nitric oxide, 105, 171
Nizoral, 60–61
Nonsurgical methods, 202–15. *See also
specific method*
Nonvellus hair, 11
Norreticuline, 214
Nutritional supplements
as cause of hair loss, 29, 31
purchasing, 182
should you take, 134–36
as treatment, 20, 23, 28, 37, 86
See also specific supplement

101 Hair Regeneration Liniment, 94
Onion, 171

Pain, 21, 23, 197
Pantothenic acid, 90, 102, 103, 142–43,
181
Parathyroid hormone related peptide
(PTHrP) antagonist, 215
Pepper plant, 95
Permanent waves, 35, 98, 116
Phenytoin, 71–73, 105
Pheomelanin, 10
Phosphorus, 146, 178

Phototherapy. *See* PUVA
Physicians, 5–6, 38–41, 200–201. *See
also specific person*
Pickart, Loren, 97–98
Pinacidil, 214
Polysorbate 20, 92
Prednisolone, 23, 49, 51
Prednisone, 49, 51, 59, 68
Preluderm, 108
Premarin, 55
Prescription drugs, 4, 29. *See also specific
medication*
Proctor, Peter H., 72–73, 75, 105, 106
Professional organizations, 220–23
Progaine Shampoo, 113
Propecia, 45, 56–57, 67
Proscar, 56
Prostaglandins, 179
Protein, 154, 178, 180
and diet and nutrition treatments,
127–29, 139, 142, 151, 153
and drug treatments, 79
functions of, 127–29
and nondrug treatments, 100, 103,
111
and telogen effluvium, 21–22
See also Amino acids
Proxiphen, 71–73, 75, 105–6
Psoriasis, 33–34, 171
Pumpkin, 167, 169
PUVA (Psoralens and Ultraviolet Light),
27, 28, 34, 59, 73, 86, 154
Pygeum africanum, 156, 167–68, 169
Pyoderma, 33
Pyroxidine. *See* Vitamin B$_6$

Radiation, 105, 154, 162
Rassman, William R., 193
Re-Mox, 82
Red pepper, 171
Renova, 79
Resins, 115, 116, 173
Reticuline, 214
Retin-A, 19, 28, 34
in combination with other agents, 67,
71–73, 75, 80, 81–82, 84, 93, 98,
105
and how it is used, 82

2019

Vellus hair, 10–11, 97
Vitamin A, 29, 79–80, 129, 137, 139, 157, 178, 181
Vitamin B$_5$. *See* Pantothenic acid
Vitamin B$_6$, 47, 90, 93, 143–44, 152
Vitamin B$_{12}$, 53–54, 135, 144, 177
Vitamin B-complex, 92, 93, 102, 103, 129–30, 134, 137, 139–44, 176, 177, 178. *See also specific vitamin*
Vitamin C, 134, 135, 137, 144–45, 150, 178, 181
Vitamin D, 137, 181
Vitamin E, 135, 137, 145, 156, 167, 181, 189

Vitamins
    as treatment, 137–45
    See also specific vitamin
Viviscal, 181–82
Volumizers, 116

Websites, 75, 225–26
Weyrich, Randall P., 200
Wigs/wiglets, 27–28, 86, 203, 204–6

Xandrox, 47, 67–68, 83–84

Zhao Zhangguang, 94–97
Zinc, 28, 47, 84, 92, 93, 105, 143, 151, 152–53

About the Author

Maggie Greenwood-Robinson, Ph.D., is one of the country's top health and medical authors. She is the author of *Natural Weight Loss Miracles, Kava Kava: The Ultimate Guide to Nature's Anti-Stress Herb, 21 Days to Better Fitness*, and *The Cellulite Breakthrough*. Plus, she is the coauthor of nine other fitness books, including the national best-seller *Lean Bodies, Lean Bodies Total Fitness, High Performance Nutrition, Power Eating*, and *50 Workout Secrets*.

Her articles have appeared in *Let's Live, Physical, Great Life, Shape Magazine, Christian Single Magazine, Women's Sports and Fitness, Working Woman, Muscle and Fitness, Female Bodybuilding and Fitness*, and many other publications. She is a member of the advisory board of *Physical Magazine*. In addition, she has a doctorate in nutritional counseling and is a certified nutrition consultant.